Ensuring value for money in health care

OF01032

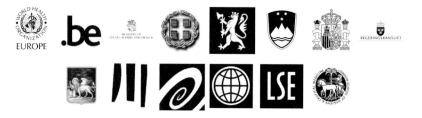

The European Observatory on Health Systems and Policies supports and promotes evidence-based health policy-making through comprehensive and rigorous analysis of health systems in Europe. It brings together a wide range of policy-makers, academics and practitioners to analyse trends in health reform, drawing on experience from across Europe to illuminate policy issues.

The European Observatory on Health Systems and Policies is a partnership between the World Health Organization Regional Office for Europe, the Governments of Belgium, Finland, Greece, Norway, Slovenia, Spain and Sweden, the Veneto Region of Italy, the European Investment Bank, the Open Society Institute, the World Bank, the London School of Economics and Political Science and the London School of Hygiene & Tropical Medicine.

Ensuring value for money in health care

The role of health technology
assessment in the European Union

Corinna Sorenson

Michael Drummond

Panos Kanavos

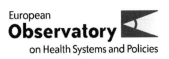

European
Observatory
on Health Systems and Policies

Keywords:

TECHNOLOGY ASSESSMENT, BIOMEDICAL – organization and administration

OUTCOME AND PROCESS ASSESSMENT (HEALTH CARE)

EVIDENCE-BASED MEDICINE

DECISION MAKING

COST-BENEFIT ANALYSIS

EUROPEAN UNION

ISBN 978 92 890 7183 3

Printed in the United Kingdom by MPG Books Ltd, Bodmin, Cornwall.

Contents

List of abbreviations

ACD	Appraisal consultation document.
Afssa	*Agence Française de Sécurité Sanitaire des Aliments.*
Afssaps	*Agence Française de Sécurité Sanitaire des Produits de Santé.*
Afsset	*Agence Française de Sécurité Sanitaire de l'Environnement et du Travail.*
ANAES	*Agence Nationale d'Accréditation et d'Evaluation en Santé National.*
ANDEM	*Agence Nationale pour le Déement de l'Evaluation Médicale.*
ASMR	*Amélioration du Service Médical Rendu.*
ATC	Anatomical therapeutic chemical.
BfArM	*Bundesinstitut für Arzneimittel und Medizinprodukte.*
BMG	*Bundesministerium für Gesundheit.*
BZgA	*Bundeszentrale für gesundheitliche Aufklärung.*
CAMTO	Centre for Assessment of Medical Technology.
CBA	Cost benefit analysis.
CBO	Dutch Institute for Healthcare Improvement.
CDC	Centers for Disease Control and Prevention.
CE	Cost-effectiveness.
CEA	Cost-effectiveness analysis.
CEDIT	*Comite d'Évaluation et de Diffusion des Innovations Technologiques.*
CEMTV	*Center for Evaluering og Medicinsk Teknologivurdering* (DACEHTA).
CEPP	*Commission d'Évaluation des Produits et Prestations.*
CEPS	*Comité Économique des Produits de Santé.*
CES	*College des Économistes de la Santé.*
CFH	*Commissie Farmaceutische Hulp* (Pharmaceutical Care Committee).
CMA	Cost minimization analysis.
CUA	Cost-utility analysis.

CVZ	*College voor Zorgverzekeringen* (Health Care Insurance Board).
DAHTA	*Deutsche Agentur für Health Technology Assessment.*
DIMDI	*Deutschen Institut für Medizinische Dokumentation und Information.*
ERNIE	Evaluation and review of NICE implementation evidence database.
EUnetHTA	European network for Health Technology Assessment.
FinOHTA	*Terveydenhuollon menetelmien arviointiyksikkö* (Finnish Office for Health Technology Assessment).
HTA	Health technology assessment.
HTAi	Health Technology Assessment International.
IHE	*Institutet för hälso-och sjukvårdsekonomi* (Swedish Institute for Health Economics.
IMOR	Institute for Medical Outcome Research.
INAHTA	International Network of Agencies for Health Technology Assessment.
Inserm	*Institut National de la Santé et de la Recherche Médicale.*
IOM	Institute of Medicine.
IQWiG	*Gemeinsamen Bundesausschuss/Institut für Qualitat und Wirtschaftlichkeit im Gesundheitswesen.*
ISPOR	International Society for Pharmacoeconomics and Outcomes Research.
ITAS	*Institut für Technik-folgen-abschätzung und Systemanalyse.*
LFN	*Läkemedelsförmånsnämnden* (Pharmaceutical Benefits Board).
MPA	*Läkemedelsverket* (Medical Products Agency).
NAM	*Lääkelaitos* (National Agency for Medicines).
NCC	National Collaborating Centre.
NCCHTA	National Coordinating Centre for Health Technology Assessment.
NHG	*Nederlands Huisartsen Genootschap* (Dutch College of General Practitioners).
NHI	National health insurance.
NHS	National Health Service (United Kingdom).

NICE	National Institute for Health and Clinical Excellence.
NoMA	*Statens legemiddelverk* (Norwegian Medicines Agency).
NSF	National service framework.
NWO	*Nederlandse Organisatie voor Wetenschappelijk Onderzoek* (Netherlands Organisation for Scientific Research).
OECD	Organisation for Economic Co-operation and Development.
PPB	*Lääkkeiden hintalautakunta* (Pharmaceuticals Pricing Board).
PCT	Primary care trust.
QALY	Quality-adjusted life year.
QIS	NHS Quality Improvement Scotland.
QUORUM	Improving the quality of reporting of meta-analyses of randomized controlled trials.
R&D	Research and development.
RCT	Randomized controlled trial.
RFV	*Riksforsakringsverket* (National Social Insurance Board).
ROHTO	*Lääkehoidon kehittämiskeskus* (Centre for Pharmacotherapy Development).
RVZ	*Raad voor Volksgezondeid & Zorg* (Council for Public Health and Health Care).
SBU	*Statens beredning för medicinsk utvärdering* (Swedish Council on Technology Assessment in Health Care).
ScHARR	School of Health and Related Research, University of Sheffield.
SHA	Strategic health authority.
SHI	Statutory health insurance.
SHTAC	Southampton Health Technology Assessments Centre.
SMC	Scottish Medicines Consortium.
SMR	Therapeutic value.
STA	Single technology appraisal.
STAKES	National Research and Development Centre for Welfare and Health.
TAB	*Büro für Technikfolgen-Abschätzung beim Deutschen Bundestag*.
TAG	Technical appraisal guidance.
TAR	Technology assessment report.
TNO	*Kennis voor zaken* (Netherlands Organisation for Applied Scientific Research).

UNCAM	*Union Nationale des Caisses d'Assurance Maladie.*
UNOC	*Union Nationale des Organismes d'Assurance Maladie Complémentaire.*
WHO	World Health Organization.
WTP	Willingness to pay.
ZonMw	*Nederlandse organisatie voor gezondheidsonderzoek en zorginnovatie* (Netherlands Organisation for Health Research and Development).

List of tables, figures and boxes

About the authors

Corinna Sorenson (MPH, MHSA) is a research officer at LSE Health, London School of Economics and Political Science and a Ph.D. candidate in the Department of Social Policy. Before joining LSE, Ms Sorenson served as a senior policy and planning analyst for the United States' Food and Drug Administration. Also, she has held various consulting positions in health policy and health economics research.

Michael Drummond (D.Phil.) is a professor of Health Economics at the University of York, Centre for Health Economics. He has undertaken evaluations over a wide range of medical fields including care of the elderly, neonatal intensive care, immunization programmes, services for people with AIDS, eye health care and pharmaceuticals. In addition, Professor Drummond has authored more than 500 scientific papers and currently serves as President-Elect of the International Society for Pharmacoeconomics and Outcomes Research (ISPOR).

Panos Kanavos (Ph.D.) is a senior lecturer in international health policy in the Department of Social Policy and Merck Fellow in Pharmaceutical Economics at LSE Health, London School of Economics and Political Science. He has acted as an adviser to a number of international governmental and non-governmental organizations including the World Bank, WHO, Organisation for Economic Co-operation and Development, American Association of Retired Persons and ministries of health in over 14 transition and developing countries.

Acknowledgements

This project was part of a year-long study: *Financing sustainable health care in Europe*. It was endorsed by Luxembourg's Ministry of Health, Sitra and the Finnish Innovation Fund.

The authors greatly appreciate the helpful comments and suggestions and time taken by the final reviewers – Dr David Taylor and Dr Frans Rutten. We are also grateful to Dr Elias Mossialos for his insightful guidance and contributions to the project.

This study was made possible with the financial support of Pfizer Inc.

Executive summary

This report addresses the concepts and controversy surrounding health technology assessment (HTA) in Europe, with a particular focus on selected Member States including Sweden, the Netherlands, Finland, France, Germany and the United Kingdom.

Extensive review of these HTA systems produced a number of key findings relevant to a wide range of stakeholders including policy-makers, HTA bodies, manufacturers, health-care professionals and patient organizations.

1. HTA plays a major part in evidence-based decision-making. Without good evidence, the uptake and diffusion of health technologies is likely to be influenced by a range of social, financial and institutional factors. This may result in suboptimal health outcomes and inefficient use of resources.

2. Innovation and the actual needs of the health-care system should be linked more closely. Products that provide the most value for investment must be identified and supported and their manufacturers rewarded with appropriate reimbursement and pricing schemes.

3. Many countries have dedicated HTA bodies, but with somewhat unclear and disparate roles and responsibilities. Groups involved in reimbursement and pricing decisions often differ from those affiliated with independent HTA assessment and clinical guidance development. Divergent processes and roles may hinder the effectiveness and efficacy of the decision-making process and lead to unnecessary duplication of efforts and resource use.

4. Most review bodies involve a range of stakeholders including physicians, health economists, pharmacists and patient group representatives. Most

agencies support some level of involvement from patients and consumers, and a greater role for industry representatives has been proposed. More stakeholder involvement is needed to improve the HTA processes and the implementation of decisions and related policy. This is true of broad HTA networks and partnerships (such as EUnetHTA) that can enhance collaboration between agencies and facilitate innovation in HTA processes and methods.

5. Some countries consider the evidence and resources required to conduct an assessment, as well as its relevance to the primary clinical and/or policy question. An assessment will not be helpful if there are insufficient data, and may delay access to new treatments. Clinical and policy relevance is especially important as HTAs are useful only if they are expected to contribute to the decision-making process.

6. Generally, HTA processes lack transparency – from prioritizing decision criteria to stakeholder involvement. More transparency is necessary to ensure an open, systematic and unbiased decision-making process.

7. There is limited information on HTA's use in identifying areas of disinvestment. More attention should be paid to identifying topics for potential disinvestment so that ineffective and obsolete products and practices do not remain in the health-care system.

8. Assessments should adopt a broader definition of value and product benefit by considering patient preferences, quality, equity, efficiency and product acceptability among a wide range of stakeholders. Further exploration to reveal how non-quantifiable factors (e.g. preferences, equity concerns) are accounted for in assessments and decision-making will enable the social implications and constraints of efficient and equitable health to be addressed effectively. In pursuit of this aim, the opinions and experiences of health professionals and individual patients are needed to understand the real-world application and use of a product.

9. Different countries have diverse technical requirements so it is important that the choice of parameters and methods is substantiated and well-documented. The model and resulting analysis should be as transparent as possible, and shared with all parties involved in its development.

10. Several technical and methodological hurdles remain. These require further investigation and include the summary measures' ability to capture other benefits important to patients and the public; generalizability of studies beyond the particular setting or country; inability to account for the opportunity costs of new and expensive technologies; and comparability of measures to ascertain patient preferences. Moreover, as the modelling of cost-effectiveness (CE) becomes more complex, more resources

should be devoted to assessing new methods and the resulting impact on uncertainty in decision-making.

11. Assessments should take account of indirect benefits and costs. It would be helpful if review bodies could agree on the inclusion of additional years of life provided by new treatments, as well as opportunity costs related to leisure activities. A better understanding of threshold values, other decision criteria and their application to the overall decision process is needed.

12. The timing of assessments can affect significantly the decision-making process and patient access. Programmes have been introduced to provide more timely information on important products. These programmes should be monitored and evaluated for effectiveness and resulting impact on access to new technologies.

13. In order to maintain the accuracy of assessments and ensure that the most valuable products are on the market, re-evaluation is key to the HTA process. Often the data needed to confirm the cost- and clinical-effectiveness of a technology can be found only after practical application in the market. This is particularly true for novel products and technologies undergoing fast-track assessment. Systems should be created to allow new clinical and health economic information to be introduced during the assessment process and following market entry. However, there must be safeguards to prevent any re-evaluation leading to inefficiency, resource burden and delayed access to treatments.

14. There is a lack of understanding and evidence on the practical application of HTA from both a process (decision-making) and an outcome (health outcomes, care delivery, costs, research innovation) perspective. More focused research is needed in these areas.

15. The scope of HTA has focused predominantly on pharmaceuticals and, less frequently, on other medical technologies such as devices. There should be further exploration of applying the principles and methods of economic evaluation to preventive measures. Additional research should establish whether (and in what circumstances) such assessments have been conducted, and identify the opportunities and challenges.

Overall, HTA can play a valuable role in health care decision-making, but the process must be transparent, timely, relevant, in-depth and usable. Assessments need to use robust methods and be supplemented by other important criteria. Maximization of HTA will enhance potential decision-makers' ability to implement decisions that capture the benefits of new technologies, overcome uncertainties and recognize the value of innovation, all within the constraints of overall health system resources.

Chapter 1

Project overview, objectives and methods

Almost all Member States have experienced exponential growth in the introduction and uptake of health technologies in recent years – new medicines and diagnostic tools, telemedicine and surgical equipment. Such innovation provides enormous opportunity for governments, providers and patients to realize improved health-care services and outcomes.

The rapid diffusion of health technologies has presented governments with unprecedented challenges to provide high quality and innovative care to meet population health needs most effectively while managing health-care budgets and safeguarding the basic principles of equity, access and choice. Consequently, governments increasingly are required to manage scarce resources strategically by investing in those services that deliver the best health outcomes. This equates to care that is affordable, effective, safe and patient-centred. Moreover, innovation is supported adequately, with sufficient market access to new treatments.

In recent years, various Member States have developed systems to identify the innovations that provide the best value. The National Institute for Health and Clinical Excellence (NICE) in the United Kingdom was the first national attempt to provide faster access to cost-effective treatments through an evidence-based review process. Review bodies, such as NICE, employ health technology assessment (HTA) to ascertain the relative costs and benefits of health technologies. The resulting evidence is used to support various forms of decision-making, such as reimbursement and pricing. In other words, this information can aid priority-setting for access to limited health-care resources. Beyond ascertaining value, increased use of HTA in this setting signals a desire for a more systematic and transparent process to allocate health-care resources.

The operations of NICE and its international counterparts have generated controversy. There are concerns regarding the methods employed during the assessment process; HTA's role and utility in decision-making and priority-setting; and the resulting impacts on health care. How are assessments prioritized and who decides? What do authorities mean by evidence? How do HTA methods differ across agencies? What, if any, impact do they have on the assessment results? Is HTA actually employed in a way that aids decision-making? What is HTA's effect on health care in terms of patient care, innovation and costs?

Spearheaded by the London School of Economics, this report aims to address the concepts and controversy surrounding HTA in Europe. The report reviews HTA organizations and processes throughout the European Union (EU) and within selected Member States including extensive case studies on Sweden, the Netherlands, Finland, France, Germany and the United Kingdom, the latter focusing on England and Wales (see Appendices).

Broadly, the report is intended to identify and address current considerations regarding HTA methodological and process issues related to the prioritization and financing of modern health care. In particular, it describes the processes and challenges for identifying and prioritizing assessments; assesses and compares current assessment methods and procedures; and highlights the barriers to effective implementation. The report also ascertains the roles and terms of engagement of key stakeholders, and captures the opportunities and challenges for the use of HTA guidance in general priority-setting, decision-making and health-care provision.

Current literature related to HTA was reviewed systematically, including peer-reviewed journals and grey literature sources. Where necessary, reports and other information sources were translated into English. Experts in HTA were consulted in order to supplement the secondary data collection and address any gaps in the evidence available.

In conclusion, the review of HTA in Europe and the overarching themes identified in the report should assist in improving the HTA process in Europe and its role in supporting value in health care.

Chapter 2

Background on innovation and HTA

Overview of innovation in health care

Health technology is an indispensable part of any nation's health-care system. During the past half-century, all Member States and several other countries have increased their technological base for health care – in knowledge and through investments in equipment, devices and pharmaceuticals. As a result, national health-care systems have become increasingly advanced as health-care delivery has introduced a range of technological innovations, such as new medicines and diagnostic tools, telemedicine and surgical equipment.

The introduction of new technologies has brought remarkable improvements. Many innovations result in applicable new therapies with significant benefits for patients including improved health, enhanced quality of life and reduced adverse or side effects. Moreover, innovations in clinical practice provide enormous opportunity for physicians and other health-care providers to improve the effectiveness, safety and quality of treatment. On a broader level, technological innovation provides governments with mechanisms to improve the quality and outcomes of national health-care objectives.

Many innovations offer significant potential benefits to patients and the health-care system, but their diffusion can prove problematic in resource-constrained health-care environments. Some innovations produce similar or improved effectiveness and quality of care at significantly lower costs; others increase overall health expenditure (Cutler & McClellan, 2001; Newhouse, 1992). Indeed, the nature and strength of the relationship between health technology and costs are complex and evolving. Moreover, demographic transition (the ageing population) and better-educated health consumers have resulted in increased demand for new medical products and services (Deyo, 2002). This technological imperative frequently is accompanied by expectations of public financing and access that will continue to exert pressure on public budgets in the context of lower economic growth. Governments must strive to attain a balance between innovation, medical progress and productivity gains through more efficient management of health-care systems.

New innovations can significantly improve clinical practice, but the rapid growth of medical technology, and the increasing volume of new knowledge from basic and applied clinical research, have made it virtually impossible for care providers to keep pace with treatment advancements. Inappropriate practices and variations in the use of new and existing technologies have encroached into health-care provision across Europe so that the most effective and efficient technologies may not always be employed. Often, inertia and reluctance to change long-standing practices and outdated education restrict the uptake of new, cost-effective interventions.

Accordingly, many EU countries face the significant policy challenge of harnessing the benefits of technology and innovation while managing health-care budgets and meeting public demand and expectations. Countries employ a wide array of approaches to control the costs of health technology and support the optimal use of such products and HTA has assumed an increasing role in national priority-setting and health-policy processes. In recent years, various Member States have developed systems to evaluate innovations – determining their relative value for investment and mechanisms for equitable and accessible treatment provision. In the United Kingdom, NICE was one of the first review bodies established to provide faster access to modern treatments through a systematic review process and to promulgate evidence-based decision-making.

HTA: overview and key objectives

HTA originated from growing concern about the expansive diffusion of costly medical equipment in the 1970s and taxpayers and health insurers' ability and willingness to fund their use (Jonsson & Banta, 1999). Moreover, greater public awareness of health-care rationing decisions and a growing consumerist position on health-care policy required more accountability, transparency and legitimacy in decision-making processes. Decision-makers needed a more comprehensive approach to set priorities and obtain maximum benefit from limited resources, without compromising the ethical and social values underpinning health systems (Hutton et al., 2006). The growth and development of HTA reflected this demand for well-founded information to support decisions on the development, uptake and diffusion of health technologies.

Since the 1970s, HTA has broadened to encompass a wide range of health technologies including drugs; medical devices; medical and surgical procedures; and the organizational and support systems for care provision (Jonsson, 2002). However, the majority of HTAs have been conducted on pharmaceuticals rather than other technologies such as medical devices and surgical procedures (Hutton et al., 2006).

On a broad level, HTA can be defined as: *The systematic evaluation of the properties, effects, and/or other impacts of health care technology* (International Society of Technology Assessment in Health Care, 2002).

More specifically, HTA involves the evaluation of an intervention through the production, synthesis and/or systematic review of a range of scientific and non-scientific evidence.[1] The type of evidence considered typically includes the safety, efficacy, cost and cost-effectiveness (CE) of a product. However, HTA is also concerned with the societal, organizational, legal and ethical implications of implementing health technologies or interventions within the health system (Velasco-Garrido & Busse, 2005; INAHTA, 2002). For example, HTA often considers health technologies' broader macroeconomic impacts on national health-care budgets; resource allocation among different health programmes; regulation; and other policy changes for technological innovation, investment, technology transfer and employment (Goodman, 1998).

In addition to ascertaining technologies of value, an effective HTA can reduce or eliminate the use of interventions that are not safe and/or effective, or have insufficient cost-benefits. HTA can also be used to identify existing technologies that may be harmful or ineffective. Less commonly, HTA can also identify underused technologies (e.g. preventive screening, smoking-cessation interventions) and the reasons for this (Asch et al., 2000; McNeil, 2001).

For a systematic review of the available evidence on a health technology(s), HTA employs a multidisciplinary framework to address four principal questions (UK National Health Service R&D Health Technology Assessment Programme, 2003).

- Is the technology effective?

- For whom does the technology work?

- What costs are entailed in its use?

- How does the technology compare with available treatment alternatives?

---

1. HTA typically entails 1) identifying the policy question, 2) systematic retrieval of scientific and non-scientific evidence, and analysis, and 3) appraisal of evidence, including judgments regarding the meaning of the evidence. The evidence and its applications then inform the decision-making process.

An HTA's principal aim is to provide a range of stakeholders (typically those involved in the funding, planning, purchasing and investment of health care) with accessible, usable and evidence-based information to guide decisions about the use and diffusion of technology and the efficient allocation of resources. In light of these objectives, HTA has been called "the bridge between evidence and policy-making", as it provides information for health-care decision-makers at macro-, meso- and micro-levels (Battista & Hodge, 1999). Decision-makers have increasingly relied on the use of HTA to support reimbursement and pricing decisions regarding existing and new pharmaceuticals. HTA also contributes greatly to the knowledge base for improving quality of care, especially by supporting the development (or updating) of clinical practice guidelines and standards for health-service provision (Zentner et al., 2005).

Without sufficient, high-quality evidence the uptake and diffusion of technologies are more likely to be influenced by a range of social, financial, professional and institutional factors. This may not produce optimum levels of health outcomes or efficient use of scarce resources.

Interface between HTA and innovation

The variety and emerging complexity of health technologies has combined with limited national budgets to produce tensions between delivering cost-effective health care and improving or sustaining a country's manufacturing and research base. The importance of achieving a balance between affordable health care and the use of innovative health technologies has increased. This requires not only consideration of the medical and economic value of a product, but also who benefits from innovations, optimal usage[2] and appropriate placement in the spectrum of care (Drummond, 2003).

HTA provides important benefits by empowering governments to make value-driven decisions, supporting innovation and providing patients and physicians with the information for making the best treatment choices.

However, HTA's effectiveness (particularly in encouraging innovation) rests on accurate assessments and the appropriate implementation and use of subsequent recommendations. HTA can encourage innovation if assessments of new technology are performed properly and consider a wide range of

---

2. Variation in uptake and diffusion can signify the sub-optimal use of technology. Excess use is signified when the costs outweigh the benefits for any additional level of technology diffusion or use. Under-use can occur when the foregone benefits outweigh the costs of additional diffusion or use. Both scenarios are sub-optimal, potentially resulting in economic costs and/or reduced health outcomes.

associated costs and benefits rather than focusing solely on acquisition costs. In particular, adoption costs need to be measured against the potential broader benefits of integrating the new technology into the health system; budget-driven constraints do not necessarily result in the selection of the most effective or cost-effective products. This may require governments to allow additional funding and flexibility between budgets so that expenditure levels are driven by value rather than arbitrary spending caps (Drummond, 2003).

As mentioned, HTA's value in encouraging innovation and value-added health care also depends on the assessment process – including when and how the review was performed and the resulting decision-making procedures. In particular, the following issues can impact on HTA's effective use for meeting key objectives (Drummond, 2006; Zentner et al., 2005; Anell, 2004; Busse et al., 2002).

- Delays in the HTA process can result in deferred reimbursement decisions, restricting patient access to treatments needed.

- Evidence requirements can be a significant hurdle for manufacturers, particularly small, innovative companies. These may discourage pursuit of breakthrough technologies.

- As HTA becomes increasingly widespread, assessments are made earlier in the technology diffusion process. This may introduce greater uncertainty into the process and the potential for innovations to appear more, or less, beneficial.

- Current assessment methodologies may limit comparability and transferability across countries and studies.

- Lack of transparency, accountability and stakeholder involvement in the HTA process can decrease the acceptance and implementation of assessment results.

- Low numbers of skilled HTA personnel and limited international collaboration between review agencies can reduce the efficiency and effectiveness of assessments.

- Separate processes and organizations for economic assessments, reimbursement/pricing decisions and practice-guideline development may hinder the effectiveness and efficacy of the overall decision-making process through unnecessary use of resources and duplication of efforts.

Decision-makers are more likely to utilize HTAs if there are established policy instruments (e.g. reports, practice guidelines) and commitments to use them effectively. Moreover, patient demand and the CE of a technology can change so it is important to review HTA recommendations on a consistent basis. This requires greater participation and collaboration among stakeholders particularly HTA personnel, government officials, the industry, health providers and patients. Without adequate input and understanding of the HTA process, stakeholders may mistrust the evidence and subsequent recommendations.

For HTA to be of optimal benefit, the assessment process needs to be linked with innovation and other aspects of policy-making – recognizing the complexities of decision-making that require consideration of subjective and normative concerns. Without these links, HTA may have limited power to inform the policy process and facilitate access to new and effective products. HTA's role in encouraging innovation and value in health care could be improved by greater understanding of the challenges inherent in the HTA process, as outlined below.

Chapter 3
HTA and decision-making in Europe

HTA dates from the late 1970s when the expansion of technology and health-care costs began to capture the attention of decision-makers (Jonsson, 2002). The introduction and subsequent growth within Europe runs alongside health policies that place greater emphasis on measurement, accountability, value for money and evidence-based policies and practices. Moreover, the advent of randomized control trials (RCTs) and subsequent availability of data; growth in medical research and information technology; and increased decentralization of health system decision-making, all contributed to an increased need for HTA activities (OECD, 2005).

In Europe, the first institutions or organizational bodies dedicated to the evaluation of health-care technologies were established in France and Spain in the early 1980s and in Sweden in 1987 (Velasco-Garrido & Busse, 2005; Garcia-Altes et al., 2004). Over the following decade HTA programmes were established in almost all European countries, either in new agencies or institutes or in established academic governmental and non-governmental units (Table 3.1). Broadly speaking, such bodies fall into two categories: (1) independent (arms-length) review bodies that produce and disseminate assessment reports on a breadth of topics, including health technologies and interventions; and (2) entities under government mandates (e.g. from health ministries) with responsibilities for decision-making and priority-setting, typically pertaining to the reimbursement and pricing of heath technologies. The latter serve an advisory or a regulatory function.

Many EU countries are supporting these efforts by investing resources in HTA and associated evaluation activities. For example, in 2007 Sweden spent around

€5.7 million on its national agency, the Swedish Council on Technology Assessment in Health Care (SBU); and the United Kingdom Department of Health allocated £35 million to NICE (SBU, 2007; United Kingdom House of Commons, 2007).

Table 3.1. *Institutions and advisory bodies responsible for HTA activities*

Country	
Austria	Federation of Austrian Social Insurance Institutions/Drug Evaluation Committee [*Hauptverband der österreichischen Sozialversicherungs träger/Heilmittel-Evaluierungs-Kommission*]
Belgium	National Institute for Sickness and Invalidity Insurance (INAMI)/ Commission for Reimbursement of Medicines [*Institut National d'Assurance Maladie-Invalidité/Commission de Remboursement des Médicaments*]
Denmark	Reimbursement Committee/Danish Centre for Evaluation and Health Technology Assessment (CEMTV)
Finland	Pharmaceuticals Pricing Board (PPB)/Finnish Office for Health Technology Assessment (FinOHTA)
France	Economic Committee on Health Products (CEPS)/Transparency Commission [*Commission de la Transparence*]
Germany	Federal Joint Committee/Institute for Quality and Efficiency in Health Care (IQWiG)/German Agency for Health Technology Assessment (DAHTA).
Italy	Committee on Pharmaceuticals/Italian Medicines Agency (AIFA) [*CIP Farmaci/Agenzia Italiana del Farmaco*]
The Netherlands	Pharmaceutical Care Committee (CFH) /Health Care Insurance Board (CVZ)
Norway	Pharmaceuticals Pricing Board (PPB)/Norwegian Medicines Agency (NoMA)
Spain	Spanish Agency for Health Technology Assessment (AETS)/Catalan Agency for Health Technology Assessment and Research (CAHTA) [*Agència de Evaluación de Tecnologías Sanitarias/ Agència d'Avaluació de Tecnología Mèdica i Reçerca*]
Sweden	Pharmaceutical Benefits Board (LFN)/Swedish Council on Technology Assessment in Health Care (SBU)
Switzerland	Federal Office of Public Health (BAG)/Confederal Drug Commission [*Bundesamt für Gesundheit /Eidgenössische Arzneimittelkommission*]
United Kingdom	NICE/National Coordinating Centre for Health Technology Assessment (NCCHTA) /Scottish Medicines Consortium (SMC)

Source: Velasco-Garrido & Busse, 2005; Zentner et al., 2005.

Additional investment brings growing recognition that the HTA process must be scientifically sound, consistent across applications, transparent and of practical use in both policy-making and health-care practice (Zentner et al., 2005; Jonnson, 2002). Further, more countries are placing greater emphasis on ensuring that the results of HTA are considered in key decision-making processes.

While European HTA agencies share many of the same basic objectives, their structures have developed separately and currently operate differently across countries. In particular, there are variations in:

- responsibility and membership of HTA bodies (governance, decision-making, priority-setting);

- assessment procedures and methods;

- application of HTA evidence to decision-making (criteria and timing of assessments);

- HTA dissemination and implementation.

Moreover, transparency and accountability are encapsulated in each of these elements of the HTA process.

The heterogeneity of HTA activities in EU countries reflects their individual health-care and political environments with differing mandates, funding mechanisms and policy-formulation roles (Velasco-Garrido & Busse, 2005; Banta, 2003). Further, HTA's use in decisions that influence the diffusion and uptake of technologies can be influenced by a myriad of factors such as income levels, reimbursement mechanisms, regulatory environments and behavioural determinants (e.g. cultural imperative for new technology). As HTA strives to connect policy and evidence, it also reflects the specific needs of decision-makers within a certain system.

Responsibility and membership of HTA entities

Most national HTA bodies can be categorized as serving either an advisory or a regulatory role in the decision-making process, depending on the intent and type of assessment required (Zentner et al., 2005). Advisory bodies, such as those in the Netherlands and Denmark, make reimbursement or pricing recommendations to a national or regional government, ministerial department or self-governing body (Zentner et al., 2005). Regulatory bodies are accountable to health ministries and are responsible for listing and pricing drugs, medical devices and other related services (Zentner et al., 2005). This is the role of HTA agencies in Finland, France, Sweden

(LFN) and the United Kingdom. Other groups mainly coordinate HTA assessments and produce and disseminate reports (e.g. Health Council of the Netherlands, Sweden (SBU)).

The mandates or responsibilities of the assessment bodies vary according to their general mission and overall policy objectives (Anell, 2004). As one component in the broader health-care decision-making process, HTA programmes typically reflect the current national policy landscape such as the need to contain costs or improve access to a given intervention or service. Economic evaluations often coincide with policies on the reimbursement, pricing and utilization of health technologies (Hutton et al., 2006). Assessments frequently assume a role in providing information to providers through practice guidelines and in supporting decisions on the investment and acquisition of health technology (OECD, 2005).

In many countries the health ministry oversees the appraisal process, although independent institutions (e.g. NICE) often are involved in managing various aspects of the assessment (Hutton et al., 2006). In many social insurance-funded health systems, the process is driven predominantly by insurance organizations (Hutton et al., 2006). However, the health ministry provides some degree of oversight even in these countries and, often, the social affairs or security ministry is involved.

Evaluation practices also differ. In general, the nature of an assessment determines which organization will conduct the evaluation. Some HTA bodies conduct assessments via in-house committees; others coordinate independent reviews by external bodies such as university research institutions or expert groups (Anell, 2004). Independent reviews present benefits and drawbacks to the assessment process. They may provide greater transparency and help to prevent or resolve disputes (Drummond, 2006; Goodman, 1998). Moreover, decentralization can widen the expertise available and bring a broader range of perspectives to the process. However, independent reviews may introduce certain methodological challenges, such as use of particular study designs (e.g. RCTs) and potential disconnections between the economic model and systematic review. A decentralization of responsibilities may also result in coordination inefficiencies; divergent agendas and methodologies; and opportunities for miscommunication between those conducting the assessment and the ultimate decision-maker(s).

HTA entities also have differing roles in the decision-making process when assessments are complete. In some countries (e.g. United Kingdom) the HTA body develops guidance and/or recommends reimbursement status; in other systems this is determined primarily by national authorities, insurance representatives or independent self-governing bodies. Moreover, some HTA committees (e.g. in Finland and France) are also involved in negotiating product prices and reimbursement with manufacturers.

All HTAs have multiple technology-related policy-making needs and perspectives across diverse stakeholder groups. Thus, HTA involves a variety of stakeholders including physicians, pharmacists, health economists, insurance and industry representatives and patients. Anell (2004) found that most reimbursement status recommendations are determined firstly by scientific members (e.g. physicians, epidemiologists) with expertise in evaluation of medicines. These decisions are corroborated by academic entities, representatives from patient organizations, health economists and (in the case of NICE) NHS managers (Anell, 2004). Participation differs across HTA bodies, although all these agencies have some level of stakeholder involvement. A recent OECD study (2005) reported that patients and consumer groups were least involved in the assessment and decision-making process. While patient perspectives were taken into account indirectly through the inclusion of safety, effectiveness and quality-of-life measures, such indicators may not adequately reflect important broader patient values (e.g. preference for one treatment, acceptability of various side effects). Measures of such preferences can play a substantial role in the assessment of new technologies and may provide useful insights into the real-world value of technologies. Greater participation of patients and consumers has been advocated in light of these potential benefits (Coulter, 2004) and some HTA systems support an increased role for patients in assessments and decision-making. NICE has established a Citizens' Council to gather public perspectives on key issues that inform the development of guidance documents. This assists the development of the social value judgments that should underpin NHS guidance.

A greater role for industry representatives has also been suggested. This is controversial as there is concern that greater collaboration between HTA entities and industry might influence the objectivity and transparency of the assessment process, particularly in the use of commercial in-confidence data. As a result, the implementation of recommendations could be hindered by appeals and general disagreement from various stakeholders.

Stakeholder involvement is generally resource-intensive, but it can improve relevancy and produce greater trust in the assessment. Accordingly, increased engagement may facilitate better overall assessments, reduce the number of appeals and improve implementation of HTA recommendations and guidance (Drummond, 2006). In particular, by playing a more integral role in the prioritization and assessment of health technologies, patients and their organizations can drive a more consensus-based policy process, especially at the macro-level of the health-care system.

Assessment procedures and methods

Assessment processes within the EU differ on a variety of issues such as topic selection, evidence/data requirements, analytical design and the methodological approach(es) employed.

Topic selection

Most HTA agencies struggle to keep pace with new technology therefore priority-setting has become an important aspect of the process to determine which products are assessed. Countries set priorities using a number of different mechanisms and criteria, through the emphasis given to different approaches (i.e. proactive, reactive, mixed) and in the process of needs identification. The topic agendas of some review bodies are set by national authorities – typically, the health minister or department of health. However, Germany and the United Kingdom have established processes for suggestions to be submitted by a wide range of stakeholders. In Germany, a board of trustees comprised of public administrators, patients and industry representatives determines HTA topics using a Delphi process (OECD, 2005). Within the United Kingdom's NHIR Health Technology Assessment Programme, advisory panels recommend priorities to the Director of Research and Development. The Scottish Medicines Consortium (SMC) aims to evaluate every new drug, formulation and indication within 12 weeks of market launch.

For review bodies responsible for reimbursement decisions, topics of assessment are based upon manufacturer submissions (a dossier of clinical and health economic evidence to support reimbursement determinations). The breadth of assessment topics varies too – some HTA agencies focus on health technologies (specifically drugs and/or devices); others attend to particular disease areas or health conditions. Several organizations conduct assessments on both products and broader health issues (e.g. SBU in Sweden). The criteria used to select topics vary across agencies, but generally include health benefit(s); impact on other health-related government policies (e.g. reduction in health inequality, improving access); uncertainty about effectiveness/CE; disease burden; potential benefits and impact of the assessment; and innovation capacity (Garcia-Altes et al., 2004; Taylor, 2001; Oortwijn et al., 1999).

Generally it is considered not cost effective to evaluate all existing technologies and interventions. Review bodies incorporate various approaches to ensure the efficiency of the assessment process in order to provide important and timely information for decision-makers. In the United Kingdom, NICE allows groups of similar technologies to be compared; the Netherlands requires certain procedures to guide proper use of drugs that are not appraised. If a drug provides several approved indications then review bodies in Sweden, the Netherlands, Norway and the United Kingdom commonly evaluate the therapy for all conditions.

Although HTA agencies cover a quite broad range of topics, some areas are studied less (e.g. low-technology and preventive interventions). This is also true for research on ineffective and obsolete technologies and interventions. Moreover, HTA bodies rarely undertake assessments to keep abreast of new areas of research and development (R&D), presumably because of limited resources (OECD, 2005). Assessments conducted earlier in a product's life-cycle have had some impact by identifying areas of uncertainty and highlighting areas for further research (OECD, 2005). Similarly, some HTA agencies have developed early-warning and horizon-scanning systems to identify new and emerging technologies that might require urgent evaluation, consideration of clinical and cost impacts, or modification of clinical guidance activities (Douw & Vonderling, 2006; Douw et al., 2003; Carlsson et al., 1998). Criteria used most often to identify candidates for early warning assessments are listed below.

- Requires attention of (or action by) politicians, hospitals and health-care administrators within certain time limits.

- Deemed cost-demanding or controversial.

- Expected to spread more rapidly than desired, according to current scientific knowledge base.

- Expected to spread more slowly than desired given technology's potential benefit.

This type of programme has been established nationally in the Netherlands, Sweden, Finland and the United Kingdom; and internationally through the European Information Network on New and Changing Health Technologies (EuroScan).[3] There is limited evidence of impacts on decision-making, but there is some concern that early assessment may be biased against new technologies, especially those of higher cost (AdvaMed, 2000).

Several studies have highlighted a lack of transparency in the topic selection process (Garcia-Altes et al., 2004; Hagenfeldt et al., 2002; Henshall et al., 1997). Many HTA organizations lack explicit processes for prioritization, including selection methods and stakeholder involvement (Garcia-Altes et al., 2004). It is important to identify the factors involved in the priority-setting process

---

3. EuroScan has 12 members (predominantly HTA agencies) in 10 countries – 2 outside Europe (Canada and Israel).

and the specific objectives as these affect the criteria for selecting assessments. Typically, there is limited mention of any political deliberation (or other normative considerations) that drives the assessment of certain technologies. Given limited resources and greater accountability, it is increasingly important to state how assessment topics are selected. A certain level of transparency is needed for an open, systematic and unbiased assessment prioritization process (Hagenfeldt et al., 2002). Perceived lack of transparency may exacerbate existing tensions about balancing access to technologies, product innovation and health expenditures between manufacturers, patients and the stewards of health-care budgets.

Evidence/data requirements

HTA systems require various types and qualities of evidence for economic evaluations (Hutton et al., 2006). Typically, manufacturers are required to submit a comprehensive summary of a product's effectiveness and CE but these data play different roles in the assessment process. In Austria, Norway and the Netherlands, HTA bodies review and validate industry data, which must be based on systematic review of available clinical and economic evidence (Zentner et al., 2005). Other organizations (e.g. NICE, SBU) perform systematic reviews in-house or through an independent evaluation group. Evidence used in these assessments may or may not include manufacturer data and generally involves broader review of various information sources. Some countries (e.g. France, Switzerland, Finland) prefer, but do not require, systematic reviews. Their assessments are based primarily on a definite number of studies (e.g. pivotal clinical trials) provided by industry (Zentner et al., 2005). Assessment of unpublished evidence (e.g. commercial in-confidence data) is considered explicitly in Austria, the Netherlands, Sweden and the United Kingdom.

Manufacturers generally submit evidence comprised of systematic literature searches and analyses of clinical and economic studies, which may or may not include modelling. The majority of HTA institutions have published guidelines to outline the methodological requirements for manufacturers and reviewers. However, such documented procedures require varying levels of detail and transparency (Zentner et al., 2005). It is typical for the pharmacoeconomic methodologies used in assessments to be described in more detail than clinical-review procedures or the evaluation of other product characteristics (Zentner et al., 2005). Most guidelines cover preferred clinical and economic evidence, comparators, specification of the outcome variable(s), sub-group analyses, costs to be included, time horizon, discounting and use of sensitivity analyses and modelling.

Differences in timing for evidence requirements have developed recently, i.e. the point at which manufacturers submit CE data . The Swedish LFN requires manufacturers to submit evidence on cost-efficacy. If this is acceptable, the product under review is allowed provisional reimbursement while CE data is collected and submitted.

Analytical design

Countries employ different analytical frameworks to guide their assessments (Hutton et al., 2006). Most evaluations assess a variety of criteria including safety and clinical effectiveness; patient need and benefit; and CE and cost of therapy (typically in relation to benefit) (Zentner, 2005; OECD, 2005; Anell, 2004). Some HTA bodies also frame the evaluation around other factors, listed and compared in Table 3.2:

Table 3.2. *Criteria for assessment*

Criteria	AT[4]	BE	CH	DE	FI	FR	NL	NO	SE	UK
Therapeutic benefit	X	X	X	X	X	X	X	X	X	X
Patient benefit	X	X	X	X	X	X	X	X	X	X
CE	X	X			X		X	X	X	X
Budget impact		X			X	X	X	X		X
Pharmaceutical/innovative characteristics	X	X				X	X			X
Availability of therapeutic alternatives	X						X		X	X
Equity considerations								X	X	X
Public health impact						X				
R&D					X					

Source: Adapted from Zentner et al. (2005) and case studies.

---

4. AT=Austria, BE=Belgium, CH=Switzerland, DE=Denmark, FI=Finland, FR=France, NL=Netherlands, NO=Norway, SE=Sweden, UK=United Kingdom.

While the particular analytical framework may depend on the specific policy question, almost all assessments consider therapeutic and patient benefit. There is also agreement that economic evaluations should be conducted from a societal perspective, taking account of costs and benefits outside the health sector rather than a narrow budget perspective on resource use (Zentner et al., 2005; Anell & Svarvar, 2000).

Assessment methods[5]

HTA uses diverse methods, but most programmes employ an integrative approach. The majority of agencies share similar methodologies and emphasize the most rigorous types of studies (e.g. use of RCTs and cost-utility analyses), but there is no standard approach for conducting assessments. Given their varying orientations, resource constraints and other factors, assessment programmes tend to rely on different combinations of methods. In particular, assessments often differ according to the (Zentner et al., 2005):[6]

- type of economic assessment required

- classification of product benefit (benefit vs. harm) – hierarchy of evidence

- choice of comparator

- specification of the outcome variable

- costs included in the analysis

- discounting

- use of CE threshold

- allowance for uncertainty

- missing and incomplete data

Type of economic assessment

In general, different countries have similar requirements for economic assessments (Zentner et al., 2005). Typically, these are guidelines that product sponsors must follow to select the type of economic assessment used in submissions. However, some countries (e.g. Switzerland) do not require

---

5. This section refers primarily to decision-making bodies that review clinical and economic evidence for product reimbursement and pricing.

6. Methodologies can also differ on sub-group analyses; time horizons; instruments to measure quality of life; and methods for calculating costs.

assessments and so no guidelines are applied.[7] Among existing guidance, CE or cost-utility analyses are most often considered appropriate analytical designs, particularly when the proposed product has significant clinical advantages over the comparator and relative benefits need to be considered against costs. Cost-utility analysis measures health outcomes in terms of quality-adjusted life years (QALYs).[8] Increasingly this has become the preferred indicator of effectiveness as it can be applied in comparisons of different therapies and, consequently, employed for priority-setting (Zentner et al., 2005). Moreover, cost-utility analysis is deemed to be associated with fewer issues than other methodological approaches, such as cost-benefit analysis. Although many assessment bodies (such as NICE) have deemed QALYs the principal measure of health outcome, still only a limited number of studies report QALYs based on the actual measurement of patients' health-related quality of life (HRQoL)[9] (Rasanen et al., 2006; Rawlins & Culyer, 2004).

Evidence to classify product benefit

Zentner et al. (2005) found that all countries consider head-to-head RCTs with a high degree of internal and external validity to be the most reliable and objective evidence of a product's relative therapeutic benefit. This also applies to systematic reviews and meta-analyses of RCTs. Moreover, the majority of review bodies favour RCTs in naturalistic settings as they reflect daily routines and country-specific care delivery. Where definitive primary studies exist, limitations must be considered. For example, elderly people and patients with co-morbidities often are excluded from clinical trials even though they are major consumers of medical products. Additionally, trials do not always collect a full range of economic data (e.g. indirect costs, health-utility measures) and the study time horizon is often too short to detect longer-term outcomes. Findings from different types of studies should be combined or synthesized to supplement available clinical data in order to formulate

---

7. In the case of Switzerland, the assessment body applies a cost-analysis approach, whereby a new product is compared with the same therapeutic category and the price is compared with those in several other EU countries (Denmark, Germany, Holland, United Kingdom, France, Austria, and Italy).

8. QALYs provide a common unit of evaluation across multiple domains, including estimating the overall burden of disease; comparing the relative impact of specific diseases, conditions, and health care interventions; and, making economic comparisons, such as the CE of different health care interventions.

9. HRQoL measures are used increasingly alongside more traditional outcome measures to assess health technologies. These capture dimensions such as: physical, social and cognitive function; anxiety/distress; pain; sleep/rest; energy/fatigue; and perception of general health. HRQoL measures may be disease-specific or general.

effective and comprehensive policies. To that end, other types of studies (e.g. case series, registries) may be preferred to RCTs for different policy questions. For instance, modelling is useful when making decisions under uncertainty.

When conducting literature searches, selecting studies and assessing the internal and external validity of clinical trials and systematic reviews/meta-analyses, all review bodies apply internationally established standards. These may be guidelines from the Cochrane Collaboration, CONSORT (consolidated standards of reporting trials), QUORUM (improving the quality of reports of meta-analyses of randomized controlled trials) or their own comparable standards (Zentner et al., 2005).

Choice of comparator

Assessments are almost always comparative – the product under review is evaluated against some specified standard of performance or other products and treatments. The choice of comparator is significant in determining the outcomes of clinical and pharmacoeconomic analyses so it is crucial to select an appropriate comparative treatment. Moreover, all relevant options must be included adequately to inform decision-making. Zentner et al. (2005) found that HTA bodies typically use two different selection procedures. Some institutions (Finland, Sweden – new pharmaceuticals only) require a product to be compared with up to three well-defined comparators; others (e.g. United Kingdom) require all relevant comparators. The most cost-effective existing therapy usually is deemed the most appropriate comparator. However, for practical considerations, HTA bodies often accept an evaluation against routine treatment or the least expensive therapy. Routine treatment for pharmaceuticals is identified by prescription or sales volume; the dosage and delivery of medication must be therapeutically equivalent. Few agencies provide information on how usual practice is determined for non-pharmaceutical treatments. Other review bodies (Switzerland, Sweden) require products to be compared to all therapies of the same therapeutic group, based on the WHO ATC (anatomical therapeutic chemical) classification system.[10] This means that only products that are reimbursed or marketed currently can be employed as comparators. An equivalent dosage form should be defined for comparator medications. France combines both approaches by considering drugs in the same therapeutic group; the most frequently prescribed, the least expensive; and the most recently listed (positive list for reimbursement).

---

10. The ATC classification system is used for the classification of drugs. It is controlled by the WHO and was first published in 1976. Drugs are divided into different groups according to the organ or system upon which they act and/or their therapeutic and chemical characteristics.

The selectors of the assessment comparator vary between countries (OECD, 2003): specified by either the assessment body (e.g. in United Kingdom) or the product sponsor (e.g. in France and Sweden). In the latter case, HTA bodies often require manufacturers and other relevant reviewers to follow specified guidelines as closely as possible when selecting a comparative treatment. Therefore, it is important that manufacturers communicate with review bodies early in the process (i.e. initial phases of study design) (Zentner et al., 2005). In the Netherlands, product sponsors often discuss the comparator a priori with the assessment body, especially in cases considering a more narrow indication than the product's label for reimbursement approval. In the United Kingdom, Portugal and Switzerland the comparator selection varies between the product sponsor and assessment entity. In most countries the government plays some role in determining the comparator selected. In the United Kingdom, the comparator increasingly is specified by the Department of Health, particularly when it recommends topics to NICE (OECD, 2003). Other review bodies, particularly NICE in the United Kingdom, consider input from stakeholders when scoping study design and comparator selection.

Selection of the outcome variable

Assessments tend to use a variety of health and economic outcome measures. As with comparator selection, the outcome measure(s) specification can influence the conclusions of the assessment. Generally, final outcome parameters that reflect long-term treatment objectives (e.g. changes in mortality, morbidity, quality of life) are preferred, but countries have differing selection procedures and specification processes. In the Netherlands, the outcome variable is outlined by the assessment body; in most countries the product sponsors are the key decision-makers for specifying this.[11] The choice of outcome variable may depend on the type of analysis to be conducted and intermediate measures are generally accepted if there is a lack of outcome data available (OECD, 2003). However, this type of study requires a strong and scientifically-based association between intermediate effect and final outcome (Zenter et al., 2005).

Costs included in the analysis

HTA bodies and governments differ on the type of costs allowed in assessments. The specification of costs typically is related to the purpose of the analysis and

11. Portugal and Switzerland do not directly specify an outcome variable.

the overall objectives of the assessment (OECD, 2003). The differences lie in the inclusion of direct and indirect costs. Some countries (e.g. Sweden) allow all costs to be included in assessments; others (e.g. the Netherlands, United Kingdom) use only direct costs.[12] There is a lack of agreement on how to account for productivity loss for indirect costs – whether a human capital or friction cost approach[13] (Zentner et al., 2005). Moreover, only some (e.g. SBU) include the costs of additional years of life due to a longer lifespan (as a result of treatment). There is also inconsistency on the inclusion of opportunity losses in changes to the quality of life related to leisure activities and time spent on household duties. Some systems (e.g. in the Netherlands) assume a societal-cost perspective despite such costs extending beyond budget constraints. However, wider costs typically are presented separately from system-related costs, therefore non-system costs may have limited direct impact on decisions.

Some countries issue guidelines. Zentner et al. (2005) found that HTA entities or governments provide guidelines on the inclusion of costs associated with other diseases resulting from prolonged life and placing utility measures against the preferences of a country's population. As data are not always transferable across countries, HTA bodies often request resource consumption and related costs based on national data. Moreover, most guidelines require a high degree of transparency in cost calculations. This entails identifying costs accurately, separating the quantity of resources consumed and the respective cost, and detailing adequately any data sources (Zentner et al., 2005; OECD, 2003).

Discounting

The use and effects of many products extend for years, especially those for chronic conditions. Where a product impacts health and treatment utilization for over one year it is considered good practice to employ discounting to assess appropriately the changes in costs and benefits over time (OECD, 2003).

Almost all HTA bodies employ discounting in assessments, typically applying an annual rate between 2.5% and 10% to both costs and benefits (Zentner et

---

12. United Kingdom includes only direct costs to the NHS and personal social services.

13. Human capital approach employs the principal that a profit-maximizing firm will employ labour up to a point when the value of the marginal product of labour is equal to the gross wage. Thus, it treats the value of each unit of time lost to ill health to be equal to the gross wage and any additional employment costs. The friction cost approach considers that workers who withdraw from work due to ill health or death will be replaced, after some period of adaptation. Even with very short-term absence, a firm can use existing capacity in its labour pool to compensate for lost work due to ill health.

al., 2005; OECD, 2003).[14] However, a discount rate of 5% is recommended to reflect a societal perspective. Either the payer or the product sponsor determines the discounting rate, according to the country. As a general rule, institutions require the discount rate to be included in the sensitivity analysis in order to determine the effects on outcomes.

Use of CE threshold

In economic evaluation, the results of a CE analysis are summarized by the CE ratio.[15] This compares the incremental cost of an intervention with the corresponding incremental health improvement. The health improvements typically are measured in QALYs gained, so the CE ratio usually is expressed as a cost per QALY gained. Treatments with a relatively lower CE ratio are considered most cost-effective. Essentially, CE ratios indicate which health technologies will provide health improvements most efficiently (Garber, 2000).

It can be problematic to interpret the results of CE analyses and, therefore, difficult to decide whether to adopt a particular treatment. As a result, a CE or willingness-to-pay threshold often serves as a general decision rule for ascertaining value for money. An intervention's CE ratio often is compared to the threshold in order to recommend inclusion or exclusion in the benefits package. Interventions with unfavourable CE ratios may be adopted if other factors (e.g. disease burden, health equity) are a consideration.

Few countries employ a formal or fixed threshold, or at least do not make this explicit. For example, NICE maintains that there is no formal threshold, but recent comments by officials and in particular guidances (e.g. on orlistat) indicate a threshold of £20 000 to £30 000/QALY (Devlin & Parkin, 2004). Rawlins and Culyer (2004) suggest that NICE bases decisions primarily on CE ratios below £20 000/QALY. However, as the CE ratio increases there is increased likelihood of rejection on the grounds of CE. Beyond NICE, the available evidence suggests that the threshold for adoption is between US$ 20 000/QALY and US$ 100 000/QALY, with thresholds of US$ 50 000 – US$ 60 000/QALY frequently proposed (Bell et al., 2006).

---

14. It is recommended that the same rate be applied to both costs and benefits but some countries use different rates (e.g. United Kingdom, Sweden).

15. The intervention under study and its alternative are denoted as 1 and 0 respectively. If C1 and C0 are the net present values of costs that result when the intervention and alternative are used, and E1 and E0 their respective health outcomes, the incremental CE ratio is simply: CE ratio=(C1-C0)/(E1-E0). This ratio, a cost per unit of incremental health effects, is used often as a measure of value.

Allowing for uncertainty

Most review bodies either conduct or require sensitivity analyses on all variables that could potentially influence the overall results, or on a subset of inputs (e.g. imprecise estimates only). This is based on the need to test or verify the robustness of assessment findings. Countries have different requirements for sensitivity analyses (e.g. application of uni- or multi-variate methods), so it is important that the choice of parameters and methods employed are substantiated and well-documented. This is especially important when assessing new technologies for which necessary data are seldom evident.

Most countries also require some form of modelling to allow for uncertainty in the variables and estimates used in assessments. Typically, models are generated by either manufacturers or the review body, sometimes both. Many review bodies develop models to substantiate the estimates provided in manufacturers' submissions and to compensate for missing or incomplete data. Increasingly, complex decision analysis models are used to ascertain CE, although these vary in quality. Many lack adequate transparency, thus making it essential to continue independent assessment of models used in economic evaluations.

Sensitivity analyses and modelling (as well as sub-group analyses) also may be used to predict the effect of certain patient characteristics (e.g. age, sex, ethnicity) on CE and equity (Michaels, 2006). Guidance from some review bodies (e.g. NICE) suggests that it might be appropriate to provide modelling of the clinical- and cost-effectiveness of treatments for subgroups of patients, but make no explicit recommendations on which variables would be considered ethical. Clear criteria for subgroup analyses, based on specific variables, could provide a framework for incorporating social values into decision-making in an explicit, transparent and consistent way.

Missing and incomplete data

Many HTA agencies face analytical challenges when dealing with data from manufacturers or sponsors. Failure to follow specific assessment guidelines may produce data that are incomplete, poorly presented or lack transparency (OECD, 2005). Moreover, sponsors may be asked to produce the same information in various formats for different countries, presumably increasing the costs of compliance and reducing efficiency.

The choice of methods can influence significantly the result of an assessment and its comparability across studies and countries. Ultimately they may impact on HTA's utility in the decision-making process (Boulenger et al., 2005). Unfortunately, there is minimal information on how agencies handle these data issues.

Application of HTA evidence to decision-making: criteria and timing of assessments

Countries employ a variety of HTA evidence to support priority-setting and other modes of decision-making (see HTA dissemination and implementation). In a comparative study by Zentner et al. (2005), all countries[16] compared a drug's therapeutic benefit[17] with available treatment alternatives. In fact, this tended to be the leading criterion for assessing a product's added value in the majority of evaluations. Health-related quality of life is deemed the most appropriate criterion for a technology's added value from the patient perspective. NICE is one of the few review bodies that has made explicit commitments to include this measure in its assessments and recommendations.

As discussed, many decision-makers do not consider CE against a fixed threshold as an absolute decision rule. Other factors are often considered beside efficacy and CE evidence:

- necessity (e.g. disease burden and severity)
- public health impact
- availability of alternative treatments
- equity
- financial/budget impact
- projected product utilization
- innovation of product (e.g. pharmacological characteristics, ease of use)
- affordability.

Rawlins and Culyer (2004) report that NICE usually requires additional justification for CE ratios over £25 000/QALY such as the degree of uncertainty; wider societal costs and benefits; and the particular features of the condition and population using the technology. The Netherlands has an ongoing discussion about adopting a decision framework based on both efficiency and equity criteria. Different thresholds would apply according to disease burden (essentially necessity) with higher CE ratios allowed for the most severe diseases.

---

16. Austria, Australia, Canada, Switzerland, France, Netherlands, Norway, New Zealand, Sweden and the United Kingdom.

17. A product is considered as having a therapeutic benefit if it demonstrates an improved benefit/risk profile compared to existing treatment alternatives. In the case of therapeutic equivalence, a drug is typically not accepted for public reimbursement or is subject to a reference pricing system. A therapy with an inferior benefit/risk profile than other viable therapies are not typically reimbursed, even in the case of lower costs.

Many countries lack transparency in their decision-making criteria. An analysis by Anell (2004) found that some review bodies rarely, if ever, outline explicitly the relative weight and importance of the criteria used for recommendations. This is especially true of societal-related and non-quantifiable considerations, such as equity and patient's quality of life. These tend to follow efficacy and CE in their importance in the overall decision process (Zentner et al., 2005). More explicit understanding of both the threshold value and the accompanying criteria and decision rules is important for a transparent and coherent decision-making process. It has also been suggested that the CE threshold should be consistent with overall budget constraints and consider equity and fairness as well as efficiency (Rawlins & Culyer, 2004; Towse, 2003).

The time required to complete an HTA can affect the application of its evidence. Specifically, there may be a conflict between ensuring comprehensive evaluations and providing timely information to decision-makers. As different countries have divergent approaches to HTA, so the time allocated and required to complete an assessment varies. More specifically, assessments range from two weeks to a few years; although the average is between three months and one year (OECD, 2005). French assessments tend to take less time (e.g. two weeks) than those in the United Kingdom (NICE) and Sweden where one-year assessments are typical (Zentner et al., 2005). The European Commission Transparency Directive (89/105/ EC) requires Member States to make decisions on reimbursement and pricing for new pharmaceuticals to be made within 180 days of marketing authorization (Zentner et al., 2005).

Some agencies have addressed the length of time required to complete assessments. Both the SBU and FinOHTA have introduced rapid reviews to facilitate the assessment process and report on emerging technologies. NICE recently instigated single technology appraisals (STAs), a new fast-track procedure to address time concerns regarding standard assessments. STAs place more emphasis on evidence submitted by manufacturers and less on extensive external review. The SMC typically applies an STA approach to its assessments, providing the NHS in Scotland with guidance based on rapid early assessment of the evidence.

Variations in the duration of assessments can be attributed to a number of factors. Depending on the overall mission, mandate and policy objectives, some agencies conduct more of an overview, where results can be delivered rapidly. In addition, some countries may have the resources to conduct primary research in situations lacking key data, but this can prolong the assessment (OECD, 2005). The rapid pace of technological development can extend or delay timelines as HTA results become obsolete or require the development of new evaluation methodologies to reflect advances. Skilled

HTA personnel may be unavailable due to resource constraints or the pace of technologies under review. The United Kingdom has striven to address this by offering training fellowships and providing a steady stream of funding for NICE appraisals. This has enabled academic units to build a critical mass of skilled personnel (Drummond, 2006).

Early appraisals can have a number of consequences. Generally, less information is available early in a product's life-cycle and these assessments rely more on manufacturers' submissions. Early review may also be less able to consider sub-groups and other restrictions, unless they are highlighted in the company submissions.

HTA dissemination and implementation

As mentioned, the results or evidence associated with HTA are used on a wide range of decisions to:

- plan resource capacities

- shape the benefit catalogue

- guide treatment provision

- inform corporate investment decisions

- identify R&D priorities and spending levels

- change regulatory and payment policy

- acquire or adopt new technology(ies).

Almost all countries require assessments to ascertain reimbursement status, although they place differing importance on the economic evidence (Anell, 2004) – France rarely considers such information when determining reimbursement status. Alternatively, some reimbursement committees may require assessments only for patented drugs and new indications, or varying requirements for different types of products such as generic drugs (Anell, 2004). Overall, health economic evidence appears to have the most impact for decisions on drugs with broad use (thus, significant potential budget impact) and when CE varies by indication or patient sub-population.

Economic evidence is also used to restrict the use of products, especially innovative and expensive technologies that may not meet firm decision parameters. Reimbursement of these can be confined to certain indications, patient populations, treatment settings and therapeutic positioning (i.e. first- or second-line therapy) (Zentner et al., 2005). In the Netherlands, expensive inpatient drugs that meet certain criteria after an initial assessment (e.g. projected sales higher than 0.5% of total drug sales in the hospital) are granted conditional reimbursement. Additional information on the drug's real-world CE is gathered during this three-year period. Reimbursement is withdrawn if further evidence does not demonstrate value for money. Conditional approvals can play an important role in minimizing uncertainty by allowing the use of technology under limited conditions. However, their utility is contingent upon gathering additional data and subsequent re-evaluation of the product (OECD, 2005). In general, technologies are reimbursed without conditions when CE and marginal therapeutic and patient benefits against competing alternatives have been established (Anell & Persson, 2005). However, some drugs for severe disease (with a small patient population) or conditions lacking treatment alternatives (e.g. orphan drugs) are covered even if they have poor CE.

HTAs also play a role in product pricing and in negotiating special agreements with manufacturers (e.g. price-volume, cash rebates) (Anell, 2004). However, the closeness of these links differs from country to country. Some countries make reimbursement decisions prior to pricing, others (e.g. Sweden, the Netherlands, Finland) consider the reimbursement and price of a product simultaneously before making a final decision. However, the different HTA schemes and cost-containment strategies adopted by countries may not have significant impacts on individual drug prices. Rather, their effect on drug costs may be more indirect, through better definition of the appropriate clinical indications for the use of treatments (Taylor et al., 2004).

Assessment results are also used to develop clinical or practice guidelines. Typically, these include recommendations on priority-setting and provide national support to assist decision-makers (e.g. policy-makers, providers) to determine effective models of treatment delivery. However, health economic evidence is currently not used optimally in developing guidelines; a minority of overall recommendations employ guidelines grounded in HTA. Berg et al. (2004) suggest that the lack of integration between HTA evidence and guideline development may be attributable to a number of factors including a disconnect between the requirements of clinical practice and data generated by HTA; the medical profession's aversion to combining economics and health; and guideline development's reliance on efficacy and effectiveness data, rather than CE. Consequently, the authors suggest that guidelines are a limited mechanism for influencing the use or uptake of new health technology (Berg et al., 2004). This is likely exacerbated by minimal coordination between guideline-producing bodies and those that set priorities and fund HTA studies, and by limited resources for their implementation. However, guideline development and HTA are beginning to converge in many countries.

Despite increasing support for the use of HTA in national priority-setting and health-care policy-making, there remains a paucity of evidence on the real-world effectiveness of economic evaluation in improving health-care planning, clinical practice, diffusion of technologies or overall health costs. The use of HTA has produced advances in technical and methodological issues, but decision-makers continue to diverge frequently from the principles of economic evaluation (Goddard et al., 2006). In addition, there is relatively weak evidence on the impact of HTA and research development, an explicit link is found in only two countries – the Netherlands and the United Kingdom (Henshall et al., 2002).

A wide range of factors may prevent decision-makers from using strict CE criteria to set priorities, or other stakeholders from using HTA products (e.g. reports, practice guidelines) in decisions on health-care provision and innovation. Goddard et al. (2006) argue that methodological shortcomings are not necessarily the main reason for lack of impact. Rather, the wider context of public-sector decision-making places political, institutional and environmental constraints on decisions. While decision-makers may value health economic information (even requesting or requiring its inclusion in the overall evidence base), other aspects of the public policy process result in sporadic and unsystematic application of HTA.

On a macro-level, HTA's orientation in the decision-making process can affect the extent to which evidence is used to inform policy and related priority-setting. In particular, countries often hold differing views on the use of HTA recommendations (Draborg & Andersen, 2006; Garcia-Altes et al., 2004). Some countries support recommendations on the grounds that experts are best suited to inform decision-making; others prefer decision-makers to be responsible for interpreting evidence and formulating conclusions to reflect political contexts, country-specific or regional conditions, or other normative circumstances (Draborg & Andersen, 2006). However, decision-makers may lack the technical expertise necessary to understand adequately the methodological strengths and weaknesses of a given assessment. Assessment bodies have done much to enhance HTA's accessibility and usability among different audiences (e.g. policy-makers, health professionals, general public), but improvements are still needed.

Although different decision structures provide policy-makers with a wide range of discretion, failure to use available HTA evidence may produce policies that lead to inefficient, ineffective and inequitable health care. Jacob and McGregor (1997) note, "however excellent an HTA may be, if it fails to be used to influence the working of the health-care system, it is without impact and must be considered without value".

 The influence of HTA depends on several other considerations, including the information needs of decision-makers; transparency of the economic evaluation and subsequent decision-making; mechanisms for disseminating decisions; and processes for monitoring and reappraising evidence (Hutton et al., 2006; Zentner et al., 2005). The usefulness of recommendations can be limited by incongruities between the societal and long-term perspective of assessments and the short-term horizon of policy-makers (the moving-target problem)[18] (Neumann, 2004). The uncertainty inherent in HTA may also hinder its use in decision-making – effective assessments identify areas of under- and over-use, and can have ambiguous effects on price determination (Crookson & Maynard, 2000). Moreover, best use of economic evaluation may be prevented by broader health-system characteristics such as decentralized management; inadequate public resources or "silo" budgeting; and existing incentives for manufacturers and academics to deliver research that is interesting rather than practical and focused (Rutten et al., 2005; OECD, 2003; Cookson & Maynard, 2000).

It has been suggested that interest groups exert significant influence on the process. Decision-making may benefit some groups at the expense of others, and particular groups may have sufficient power to affect government choices (Goddard et al., 2006). The Dutch Council for Public Health and Health Care (RVZ) (2006) noted that, thus far:

> …decisions regarding payment or non-payment for medical treatment are only based on a limited degree on 'hard' factors, such as cost-effectiveness, and much more on less transparent considerations, as a result of pressure by lobby groups, such as consumer organizations, the media, and so on. This means that limits are indeed being set at present, but on an ad hoc and somewhat random basis. The result is that the available resources are not being deployed as efficiently as possible.

However, effective implementation of HTA requires the involvement of key stakeholders such as providers and patients. A recent OECD study found stakeholder acceptance to be one of the key determinants of whether decisions are actually put into practice within health systems (OECD, 2005).

It is difficult to assess in practice HTA's ability to maximize health for a given budget. In fact, few countries have formal processes to measure the impact of HTA. The long-term nature of some effects of HTA (e.g. changes in expectations and behaviour patterns of users) and the fact that economic evaluation is just one of many factors influencing policy and practice decisions are obstacles to measuring the impact of assessments (Hailey et al., 1990).

---

18. Often there is the possibility that by the time an HTA has been conducted, reviewed and disseminated, its findings may be outdated by changes in a technology, how it is employed or its technological alternative for a given problem.

A clear and well-communicated decision-making process must be in place before recommendations can be implemented. Lack of a defined process can create doubts about the legitimacy of decisions and make them less likely to be supported by stakeholders. This may increase the risk of appeal procedures (Drummond, 2006; Neumann, 2004). Furthermore, ill-defined decision-making processes may prevent the producers of evidence delivering timely and relevant advice. A clear decision-making process requires identification of an assessment framework that aligns incentives with evidence and health system objectives.

Improved transparency and effective dissemination of recommendations also depends on the methods used for implementing decisions (Box 3.1).

Box 3.1. Methods for disseminating and implementing recommendations

- Coverage/reimbursement policy
- Formulary restrictions
- Medical audit/peer review
- Clinical guidance
- Accreditation
- Standards
- Media campaigns
- Conferences/workshops
- Professional education
- Web sites and newsletters

HTAs with well-chosen and appropriate policy instruments; a prior commitment to use assessment findings; stakeholder involvement; and real-world applicability (e.g. not too narrowly focused) of the resulting decisions are more likely to influence practice and, ultimately, health outcomes (OECD, 2005; Henshall, 2002). Clinical guidance documents on the use of health technologies are more likely to be adopted when there is strong professional and financial support, in organizations that have established systems for tracking implementation, and when they reflect the appropriate clinical context (Sheldon et al., 2004).

Recommendations by HTA agencies and any resulting decisions must be reviewed and re-evaluated regularly to avoid the moving-target problem. This applies to new technologies and to those already on the market. Some countries (e.g. Finland, France, United Kingdom) have a more structured process for reappraisals and conduct re-evaluations at fixed or variable intervals. Others (e.g. Austria, Switzerland) initiate reviews if new characteristics of products emerge (e.g. new or broader indication) or new or better clinical and/or economic evidence becomes available (Zentner et al., 2005).

National and international collaboration is one final area that may improve HTA's impact on decision-making. Improved cooperation between assessment groups can facilitate the development of methodologies; enhance the transferability and transparency of HTA results and recommendations; and potentially improve the efficiency and accountability of the process itself. The variety of HTA activities and multiplicity of customers also necessitate strong collaboration within and between agencies and different entities dealing with HTA. Several countries have increased collaboration by creating standardized assessment guidelines or standards; convening periodic meetings to discuss assessment issues; devising new channels to encourage communication among national HTA groups; and strengthening the role of international assessment organizations (e.g. Health Technology Assessment International – HTAi) operating at the global level (OECD, 2003). Most countries engaged in HTA activities are involved in one or more international organizations. The European Network for HTA (EUnetHTA) was formed recently to connect public national/regional HTA agencies, research institutions and health ministries, in order to enable effective exchange of information and support Member States' policy decisions. EUnetHTA represents 59 partner organizations, including FinOHTA, IQWiG, DAHTA, the National Coordinating Centre for Health Technology Assessment (NCCHTA) and the SBU.

Overall implementation of HTA could be enhanced by ensuring that it adapts to the policy question and needs of decision-makers. Timely, methodologically sound evidence should be available in line with decision priorities, recognizing the various dynamics of health technology markets and the public policy process. Indeed, responsibility for achieving better alignment between assessments and stakeholder needs requires collaboration and effort from users and producers. Increasing engagement of key constituencies (e.g. patients, providers, industry) will make decision-making processes more acceptable, relevant and transparent.

Chapter 4
Conclusions

Without high-quality evidence, the uptake and diffusion of technologies is likely to be influenced by a range of social, financial and institutional factors. This may not produce optimum health outcomes or efficient use of limited resources. HTA is a significant aid to evidence-based decision-making, but it must address the challenges of delivering timely and relevant information that reflects adequately the dynamics of technology and the health-care system in order to provide the information needed for effective decision-making and priority-setting.

There is a particular need for greater correspondence between the actual requirements of the health-care system and innovation. Products that provide the most investment value must be identified and supported and their manufacturers rewarded with appropriate reimbursement and pricing schemes. Overall, the benefits of health technologies must be harnessed while simultaneously managing health-care budgets and protecting the basic principles of equity, access and choice.

This report identifies several key issues that affect HTA's usefulness in supporting effective and efficient decision-making and value-added health care.

- Many countries have several bodies dedicated to HTA, with somewhat unclear and disparate roles and responsibilities. Lines of division typically separate entities involved in reimbursement and pricing decisions from those engaged in independent HTA assessment and clinical-guideline development. Divergent processes and roles may hinder the effectiveness and efficacy of the decision-making process and lead to unnecessary resource use and duplication of efforts.

- Most review bodies involve a range of stakeholders including physicians, health economists, pharmacists and patient group representatives. However, patients and consumers – the ultimate end-users of a given technology – have limited roles in most agencies. NICE has sought to enhance their role in assessments and subsequent decision-making by establishing a Citizens Council that allows these stakeholders to comment on priorities and recommendations. A greater role for industry representatives has been proposed; both NICE and the LFN consult with industry throughout the assessment process. Overall, greater stakeholder involvement is needed to improve the implementation of decision and policy and manage uncertainty while simultaneously allowing access to safe technologies.

- While the processes for prioritizing assessments differ between countries, the majority of agencies select topics based on health benefit; disease burden; technology relevance and costs; and societal and ethical considerations. Some countries also consider the evidence and resources required to conduct an assessment, as well as relevance to the primary clinical and/or policy question. This is important as HTAs are useful only if they are expected to contribute to the decision-making process. Moreover, if the necessary data and resources are insufficient or lacking, the assessment will not be helpful and may even delay access to new treatments.

- There have been improvements in topic selection, but generally the process lacks transparency – from prioritizing decision criteria to stakeholder involvement. A greater level of transparency is necessary to ensure an open, systematic and unbiased decision-making process.

- Most agencies focus on assessments of new technologies. More attention to identifying topics for potential disinvestment will ensure that ineffective and inefficient products and practices do not remain in the health-care system. This will help to support real innovation.

- Most agencies have published guidelines to steer evidence collection and the review process. The majority of guidelines cover similar requirements (e.g. comparators, costs to include), but some important differences can impact assessments.

(1) Countries have different evidence requirements. Some differences are attributable to the particular agency's overall mission and mandate. For instance, groups involved in reimbursement and pricing decisions tend to rely on manufacturers' data, which may or may not include systematic reviews of the evidence.

(2) Most countries use QALYs as the preferred indicator of effectiveness for their cost-utility analyses. However, only a few studies use QALYs to measure

patients' health-related quality of life, so there may not be sufficient evidence of these benefits.

(3) Most countries rely on (and prefer) head-to-head RCTs to demonstrate a product's relative benefit. Although considered the most objective type of evidence, they have limitations when ascertaining product value. Assessments should not only include observational studies and other important evidence, but also adopt a broader definition of value and product benefit by considering patient preferences, quality, equity, efficiency and product acceptability among a wide range of stakeholders. The opinions and experiences of health professionals and individual patients are needed to understand the real-world application and use of a product. Except those in the United Kingdom, Sweden and the Netherlands, few agencies consider equity issues explicitly in assessments and subsequent decision-making.

(4) Assessments should take account of indirect benefits and costs. Several countries include indirect costs in analyses and a broader societal perspective, but there is a general lack of agreement on how to account for productivity losses – whether by friction cost or a human-capital approach. The results of assessments may differ significantly according to the method used. In addition, it would be helpful if review bodies could agree to include additional years of life (due to longer lifespan gained from treatment) as well as opportunity costs related to leisure activities. Evaluations should account for other indirect benefits such as reductions in treatment costs and availability of treatment alternatives in a particular therapeutic market.

(5) Few countries apply a fixed or formal CE threshold, although often the evidence suggests a range of thresholds. While the threshold can indicate an organization's or country's willingness to pay, other factors are often considered. However, these criteria and accompanying decision rules are rarely explicit. This requires better understanding of threshold values, other decision criteria and their application in the overall decision process.

(6) Most countries require sensitivity analyses and/or modelling to allow for uncertainty in the variables and estimates used in assessments. As different countries have different requirements, the choice of parameters and methods must be substantiated and well-documented. This is particularly true when more than one entity is involved in the development and analysis of models. The model and resulting analysis should be as transparent as possible, with collaboration and information exchange between all involved parties. In addition, the validity of evaluations will become more difficult to ascertain as CE modelling becomes more sophisticated. Consequently, more resources should be devoted to assessing new methods of modelling and the resulting impacts on uncertainty in decision-making.

- Technical and methodological hurdles remain despite ongoing improvements. These require further investigation and research and include: summary measures' ability to capture other benefits important to patients and the public; generalizability of studies beyond a particular setting or country; inability to account for the opportunity costs of expensive, new technologies; and comparability between health state elicitation instruments.

- The timing of assessments can significantly impact the decision-making process and patient access. There has been a general trend towards setting up new mechanisms for issuing guidance on new technologies prior to, or immediately after, market entry. Several agencies have developed early-warning or horizon-scanning systems to identify new and emerging technologies that might require urgent evaluation. In addition, NICE recently introduced STAs as a fast-tracking tool for assessments. These types of programmes have been introduced to provide more timely information on products deemed of policy, clinical or cost importance. While still relatively new, these programmes should be monitored and evaluated for effectiveness and their resulting impact on access to new technologies.

- Assessments are beneficial only if they are employed to support decision-making. The involvement of relevant stakeholders facilitates the acceptance and implementation of decisions. Moreover, a transparent and well-communicated decision-making process is vital to ensure legitimacy and acceptance of subsequent recommendations. The availability of relevant policy instruments and collaboration between national and international HTA bodies also facilitate effective and efficient implementation of decisions. Initiatives such as EUnetHTA should be supported to enhance the transferability, efficiency and accountability of the HTA process.

- Re-evaluation is a key component of the HTA process – maintaining the accuracy of assessments and ensuring that the best products are on the market. It allows for consideration of new data and accounts of uncertainty during the initial valuation process. Often, the data needed to confirm the cost- and clinical-effectiveness of a technology can be truly ascertained only after practical application in the market. This is particularly true of novel products and technologies undergoing early or fast-track assessment. Systems should be created to allow for the introduction of new clinical and health-economic information during the assessment process and following market entry. However, safeguards must be introduced against inefficiency, resource burden and delayed access to treatments. It will be useful to monitor approaches such as that of the LFN in Sweden. This allows products on to the market on a provisional basis while CE data are collected to support manufacturers' submissions.

Some limitations and areas of recommended future inquiry raised by current evidence deserve mention. There is a lack of understanding (and evidence) about HTA's real-world impact on decision-making processes and (more broadly) health outcomes, care delivery, health-care costs and research innovation. Several challenging questions remain about the circumstances surrounding the practical use of economic evidence in decision-making and priority-setting. Exactly when is it used? How are criteria operationalized and how are they weighted against the broad spectrum of decision factors? For a given disease area or public health problem, has HTA appropriately and accurately identified interventions that have led to improved health outcomes? Has HTA produced better managed health-care budgets or a decrease in health-care costs? Does HTA provide sufficient incentives to facilitate innovative R&D? Conversely, has this "fourth hurdle" in the reimbursement process deterred manufacturers from investing in new and innovative therapies? How can HTA be applied more broadly? Clearly, these questions need more focused research. Greater efforts should be made to set up a formal evaluation component within the HTA process. The impact of economic evaluation can be enhanced only by securing a better understanding of the decision-making process and the practical application of HTA.

There is limited information on HTA's use in identifying areas of disinvestment. This requires more research to identify ineffective and obsolete technologies and interventions. Assessment methodologies have advanced significantly, but there is limited knowledge of, or publicly available information on, how non-quantifiable factors are considered in the HTA process – particularly equity concerns. It is necessary to ascertain how these issues are addressed, in both assessments and subsequent decision-making, in order to address effectively the social implications and constraints of efficient and equitable health care.

There is also a lack of research on the systematic assessment of public health interventions, especially those focused on prevention. HTA to date has focused on pharmaceuticals and, less frequently, other medical technologies such as devices. There should be further exploration of applying the principles and methods of economic evaluation to preventive measures in order to facilitate a more evidence-based approach to important population health issues (e.g. obesity, smoking). Given the limited evidence on the economic evaluation of public health interventions, more research should be funded to identify completed assessments and what they have revealed.

Finally, stakeholders in the HTA process play an important yet poorly understood role. Existing evidence shows that stakeholder involvement can lead to greater transparency, relevancy and acceptance of decisions. However, there has been little attention to how they are involved in the assessment process and how and when their perspectives are considered. As one of the guideposts for successful implementation, this requires additional enquiries on the role and influence of various stakeholders, especially patients and consumers.

In conclusion, HTA plays a valuable role in health-care decision-making when the process includes transparency, timeliness, relevance and usability. Moreover, assessments must employ robust methods and be supplemented by other important criteria in the decision-making process. Decision-makers who maximize HTA's potential will improve their ability to implement decisions that capture the benefits of new technologies, overcome uncertainties and recognize the value of innovation within the constraints of overall health system resources.

APPENDICES: select country case studies

Appendix 1. Sweden

Overview of health-care and reimbursement systems

The availability of adequate health and medical care is a central tenet of the Swedish welfare state. The 1982 Health and Medical Service Act sets out equal access to health services and good health as cornerstones of the Swedish health-care system[19] (Glenngard et al., 2005). Three primary principles underpin the provision of health and medical care in Sweden, in the following order of precedence:

1. human dignity

2. need and solidarity

3. CE.

These priorities are reflected in national regulations and law.

Health and medical care is considered a public sector responsibility,[20] with public ownership and political control organized on three levels – national, regional and local (municipalities). Overall goals and policies are established at national level by the Ministry of Health and Social Affairs and the National

---

19. According to the Act , "…every county council shall offer good health and medical services to persons living within its boundaries… and promote the health of all residents".

20. Approximately 80% of health services in Sweden are considered a public sector responsibility.

Board of Health and Welfare. County councils[21] form the basis of the health-care system, responsible for the provision of health care as required by the Health and Medical Service Act. Specifically, county councils plan the development and organization of services according to the needs of their populations and publicly financed health care (Glenngard et al., 2005). Accordingly, councils have a high degree of autonomy and decision-making power for a wide range of activities, including major investments in facilities, new technologies, user fees and private practitioners' services (Carlsson, 2004). The municipalities (289) are responsible for long-term care of the elderly (i.e. nursing homes and housing) and social services (Glenngard et al., 2005; Carlsson, 2004). Moreover, local government has authority to introduce policies concerning choice of providers, contracting, hospital mergers, new primary-care models and integrated care.

The Swedish health system is funded primarily through taxation. Both county councils and municipalities levy proportional income taxes (typically around 30%) on the population. These are used in conjunction with state grants and user fees to cover health-care services (Glenngard et al., 2005; Carlsson et al., 2000). The high tax rate allows for public financing of most health-care services, including the majority of drug costs.

Central government is characterized by decentralized power and responsibility for health care. However, it guides the overall direction of the system by ensuring that health care is efficient and in accordance with national objectives and the goals of social welfare policy. Actual responsibility for implementing and administering government policy lies with a number of central administrative bodies. The Medical Products Agency (MPA) oversees the distribution, regulation and financing of pharmaceuticals. It has particular responsibility for regulatory control of drugs and other related products, including providing information about medicines and approving clinical trials and licences (Glenngard et al., 2005; Carlsson et al., 2000). The Swedish national health insurance system finances care under the auspices of the National Social Insurance Board (RFV), which also oversees price negotiations for pharmaceuticals (Carlsson et al., 2000).

Historically, a new therapy would be registered and priced by the RFV and the product sponsor following an MPA review of safety and efficacy. Once a price was established, drugs were reimbursed through the health insurance system, typically without evaluation of clinical value or relative CE (Carlsson,

---

21. There are 21 county councils in Sweden, including 3 large regions (Stockholm, Skane, West), each has over 1.5 million residents (Carlsson, 2004).

2004). However, the mechanisms related to the distribution, pricing and reimbursement of drugs underwent widespread scrutiny as drug costs escalated during the 1990s. Further, there was a focus on the need for more explicit priority setting, increased transparency for access and quality, and greater opportunity for patients to influence decision-making. In the late 1990s and early 2000s, Sweden passed several reforms in an attempt to curb increasing expenditure on pharmaceutical products (Glenngard et al., 2005) (Fig. A1.1). The New Pharmaceutical Benefits Reform (2002) was passed to increase the cost-effective use of public-financed pharmaceuticals and to ensure equal drug benefits throughout the country. This established a new independent governmental agency to meet this end and to increase the transparency of explicit priority-setting processes (Pharmaceutical Benefits Board, 2002). The introduction of the Pharmaceutical Benefits Board (LFN) produced significant changes in the pricing and reimbursement of drugs in Sweden – decisions are based on CE data rather than reimbursed automatically within the benefit scheme (Anell & Persson, 2005).

Fig. A1.1. *Principal reforms in the Swedish pharmaceutical market.*

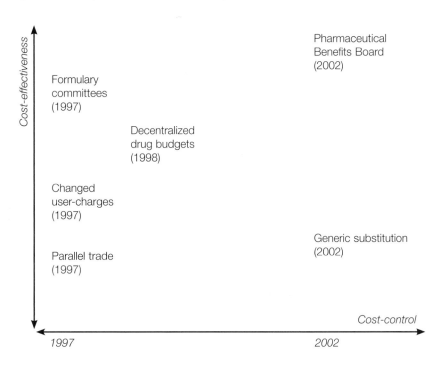

Source: Adapted from Anell and Persson, 2005.

The LFN's principal aims are to determine if a new drug (or other medical product) should be included in the positive list for public reimbursement (i.e. the Drug Benefit Scheme), and to negotiate with manufacturers to set the price of the product (Zentner et al., 2005). Moreover, the LFN is responsible for reviewing listed drugs[22] to ascertain whether they meet certain criteria outlined by the 2002 reform.[23] A five-year time frame was set for review of approximately 2000 drugs (Zentner et al., 2005) (see following section: HTA process and procedures).

The LFN comprises one director and ten members; announced by the government every five years (Zentner et al., 2005). The Swedish Government appoints four members with special expertise in health economics; the provincial parliament appoints four members with medical expertise. The other two members are representatives of consumer and patient groups. The review process is conducted by a group consisting of certain LFN members (e.g. pharmacists, health economists), as well as two to four external medical experts, typically physicians and nurses.

In addition to central governmental structures, country councils have local formulary committees that are responsible for recommendations on the use of pharmaceuticals (Glenngard et al., 2005).

HTA governance and organization

Sweden has been at the forefront of HTA within the EU and was one of the first countries to assess health technologies in the early 1970s (Carlsson, 2004). The Swedish Council on Technology Assessment in Health Care (SBU) was established in 1987.[24] As the leading HTA entity, the SBU's primary objective was to improve the efficiency and equity of access to, and use of, technologies proven safe and effective – not cost-containment (Carlsson et al., 2000). As the focal point for HTA activities in Sweden, the SBU's remit is to provide central government and health-care providers with information on the overall value of medical technologies, especially new therapies, from medical, economic, ethical and social points of view (Glenngard et al.,

---

22. Drugs with new strengths do not require reviews.

23. Since October 2002, any prescribed drug that qualifies for a subsidy is required to be exchanged for the cheapest comparable generic alternative available at the pharmacy. The MPA determines which drugs are exchangeable.

24. The SBU was formally established as a national agency in 1992, following an independent evaluation required by the central government. This resulted in a significant increase in the SBU budget and demand for systematic reviews and other HTA activities.

2005; Carlsson, 2004). Specifically, the SBU reviews the benefits, risks and costs of health technologies used in health-care delivery (Glenngard et al., 2005). It also assists in identifying areas requiring further research. The SBU Board comprises representatives from key health-care organizations who set assessment priorities and organize HTA projects. A multidisciplinary team of leading experts from Sweden and abroad is recruited for each assessment project. Further, a number of county councils have formal links with the SBU; a few finance local HTA units. The SBU recently established a formal agreement with the National Board of Health and Welfare and the MPA aimed at improving cooperation within HTA activities in Sweden and the dissemination of guidelines and information.

There are several other health assessment bodies at both regional and local levels.[25]

- *Centre for Assessment of Medical Technology* (CAMTO) in Orebro. Established in 1999 with the primary objective of promoting HTA at the local level. Comprises a network of clinicians, experienced practitioners and qualified researchers. External experts often serve as consultants on study design issues and dissemination strategies. Overall, CAMTO conducts primary research, disseminates HTA results locally and proposes new projects to the SBU.

- *Institute for Health Economics* (IHE) in Lund. Established in the mid-1970s to perform economic evaluations and other related policy analyses. Also undertakes independent method development; participates in scientific conferences/meetings; collaborates with external researchers on various health economics projects; and coordinates commissioned courses and seminars. Most IHE projects are funded directly by stakeholders in the health-care sector and most findings are published in scientific periodicals by external publishers and other institutions.

- *Centre for Health Economics, Stockholm School of Economics.* Well-respected international HTA body that collaborates on several SBU projects.

- *Center for Medical Technology Assessment* (CMT) in Linköping. Performs assessment studies of medical technology from various perspectives (e.g. social, economic, ethical, medical). Majority of activities commissioned and funded by health-care providers, international research foundations and commercial clients.

---

25. Although there are other HTA bodies, this case study focuses on the SBU – the leading HTA agency in Sweden.

HTA process and procedures

There is not enough time or resources available to review all existing technologies, so the most policy-relevant technologies are prioritized for assessment. The SBU initiates this process by submitting an annual report to the government. This reviews work accomplished, plans for future work and evaluated and projected impacts (Carlsson et al., 2000). In turn, the Ministry of Health notifies the SBU about national objectives and the annual budget. National objectives typically are determined by the Ministry of Health, Swedish Parliament and various health-care organizations, and tend to focus on broad health issues. Individuals, predominantly from the health field, also nominate topics for assessments.

Subsequent to topic nomination, the SBU sets priorities for assessment based on a two-fold process. First, an internal filtering process is used to establish all possible assessment options by scanning different fields of interest and devising a list of topics for discussion by project coordinators and the SBU executive committee (Carlsson, 2004). Second, the SBU Board receives a condensed list containing proposals ranked and selected for pilot review. Pilot studies (typically entailing an extensive literature search, the Cochrane database and other sources) ascertain whether there is sufficient existing scientific evidence to warrant a full review. The SBU Board makes a final decision based on the following selection criteria (Carlsson, 2004; Carlsson et al., 2000).

- Health impact – topic should have significant impact on health outcomes such as mortality and morbidity.

- Breadth of health problem – topic must relate to a common health problem, with significant economic consequences for society.

- Societal and ethical considerations – topic may have ethical and social implications; be controversial; or of great concern to the broader public.

- Professional or organizational justification – topic's perceived importance should be demonstrable from an organizational or professional perspective (i.e. technology may have potential significantly to alter clinical practice).

- Methodological requirements.

- Cost of technology – especially if overall value is in question.

- Technological relevance – may be obsolete product but still used extensively.

Following a positive final determination the Board appoints a project chairman and an appropriate project team.

Since the 1990s, the SBU has relied predominantly on systematic reviews as the fundamental assessment methodology rather than performing original research. Each project team, normally 10 members, establishes criteria and conducts comprehensive assessments by systematically searching, selecting, reviewing and evaluating available research findings. Typical criteria are time to follow-up, participant drop-out rates and relevant end points (Carlsson, 2004). Every study that meets the basic criteria is reviewed by at least two members of the project team and classified into one of three quality and relevance levels – low, medium and high. As well as clinical aspects (e.g. preventive, diagnostic, treatment), each assessment contains an economic and, frequently, an ethical and social component. SBU project teams typically employ guidelines or standardized checklists to direct the review process for economic evidence (Carlsson, 2004; Drummond et al., 1996). These outline different evaluation criteria including: study design (e.g. clear relevance and associated hypotheses, analysis perspective); selection of comparator(s) (rational and transparent justification for selection); type of economic analysis (e.g. CE, cost-benefit) and rationale for selected methodology(ies); breadth and quality of effectiveness data; benefit measurement and valuation (appropriate outcome measures); costing (methods of estimation and reporting of quantities and prices); modelling (with clear description and justification, including key input parameters); discounting (time horizon and discount rate provided); allowance for uncertainty (sufficient consideration of uncertainty related to data inputs, extrapolation/modelling, analytical methods); presentation of study results (availability of disaggregated data, information on any incremental and comparative analyses, clear presentation of findings).

Once the evidence has been reviewed systematically and results assembled, the draft report is reviewed by selected committee members and then by the SBU Board and a Scientific Advisory Committee. The Board gives final approval in a summary document and list of recommendations. A comprehensive final assessment report, a Yellow Report, is then published and disseminated. HTA findings are monitored and updated as necessary.

The scope of assessments can range from expansive – covering broad health problems such as obesity – to more narrow evaluations of single interventions such as Magnetic Resonance Imaging (MRI) (Carlsson, 2004). The wider-ranging reports (characterized by the Yellow Reports described) were characteristic of evaluations in the 1990s and can take several years to complete. This lengthy duration may render the results irrelevant to the needs of policy-makers (Carlsson, 2004). In response to this concern the SBU instituted SBU Alert in 1997. This provides early identification and assessment of new technologies through relevant, policy-oriented information on their potential impact in order to optimize their diffusion (Carlsson, 2004). The

Alert promotes communication on important health issues between experts and non-experts. It aims to identify relevant health technologies and assess their relative value and impact on care delivery, and to ascertain areas for additional research. Based within the SBU, the Alert is a joint effort between the SBU, MPA, National Board of Health and Welfare and the Swedish Association of Local Authorities and Regions (SBU, 2006).

The Alert programme has a slightly different assessment process for early reviews. New topics are identified via scientific sources; search of the EuroScan database for information from other early warning units; and requests from medical experts and policy-makers (Carlsson, 2004). Potential proposals on new technologies are reviewed by staff and decided by the Board, employing the following selection criteria (Carlsson, 2004):

- significant economic consequences
- ethical implications
- considerable impact on health-care organization
- potential for medical breakthrough
- concerns significant patient population or affects a common health problem.

Typically, an early review assessment involves one external expert and one SBU reviewer. Information is collected and synthesized on the new technology and its associated effectiveness, risks, CE, ethical and social concerns and organizational impact. The SBU collaborates with experts to produce brief assessments that provide timely information to key stakeholders. These Alert Reports are published on the Internet for review and comment and revised accordingly. A network of approximately 4000 health-care professionals receives this information (Carlsson, 2004).

SBU also develops special topic papers (White Reports) that explore health-care problems or interventions that may require assessment (SBU, 2006). These serve as starting points for future systematic literature reviews and are reviewed by project groups and external experts only.

Since 2005, SBU has published more than 120 reports, including the following topics:

- stroke (1992)
- MRI (1992)
- prostate cancer screening (1995)
- oestrogen treatment (1996)

- smoking cessation methods (1998)

- back pain (2000)

- colorectal cancer screening (2002)

- obesity (2002)

- moderately elevated blood pressure (2004).

The LFN establishes appraisal priorities by sales volume in each therapeutic group. The Board considers the three basic principles that underpin the Swedish health-care system for all related decisions for each appraisal. In addition, decisions are based on both the CE and the marginal utility of products (Anell & Persson, 2005). In April and June 2004, the LFN published *Working guidelines* for the evaluation of already-approved drugs as well as general pharmacoeconomic guidelines.

The LFN primarily reviews clinical and economic evaluations submitted by manufacturers as part of their application packages for reimbursement for specific products, rather than particular medical indications (Zentner et al., 2005; Glenngard et al., 2005) (see Table A1.1). However, the Board can make exceptions and authorize reimbursement for a certain indication or patient sub-group. It may allow reimbursement for a more limited indication than a drug's original MPA licence for market approval. Before any final recommendation, however, manufacturers and the Swedish Parliament may make submissions to the LFN. Any manufacturer dissatisfied with the final decision can appeal to an independent court (Anell & Persson, 2005). Between 2002 and 2005, the LFN reviewed and made decisions on 107 products; the majority approved for unconditional reimbursement (Anell & Persson, 2005).[26]

HTA dissemination and implementation

The SBU's findings are disseminated through a variety of channels, depending on the relevant target group(s). These include health-care managers, patients, purchasers, quality-improvement teams, drug-review committees and other decision-makers at regional, county and municipal levels. The delivery mechanisms include the SBU newsletter (over 100 000 copies per issue) and web site; medical and academic journals; and professional conferences, seminars and training sessions. At regional level, the SBU collaborates with the National Board of Health and Welfare, MPA, LFN and a range of professional health-care and insurance organizations to implement the findings

---

26. There may be other products that were not included on the LFN web site; moreover, sponsors may withdraw submissions before the LFN decision is made.

of SBU assessments. Effective dissemination and implementation require local involvement, so the SBU has organized a nationwide network of various experts. These act as local ambassadors to initiate and promote local (frequently regional) efforts to help ensure that decision-makers use reports and that findings are applied in clinical practice (SBU, 2006; Carlsson et al., 2004).

The findings of SBU assessments and manufacturer-sponsored economic evaluations (in the case of the LFN) are used to inform decisions and priority-setting activities, primarily for reimbursement, pricing and clinical policy and practice via the promulgation of guidelines. The LFN typically makes decisions on including or excluding new drugs in the benefit package within a 12-month review process. Since the end of 2003, the LFN has made reimbursement decisions on therapeutic groups including migraine medications, antacids, antihypertensives, asthma medications, antidepressants, cholesterol-lowering medicines, pain relief and anti-inflammatory medications and antidiabetics (Anell & Persson, 2005). Assessments of medications to treat prostate disease, incontinence and gynaecological problems are planned (Zentner et al., 2005). In general, drugs are reimbursed without conditions when CE and marginal benefits have been established from comparisons (Anell & Persson, 2005). However, some drugs with poor CE are covered if the disease is severe (with a small patient population) or there is a lack of treatment alternatives (e.g. orphan drugs).

In addition to other central government and assessment bodies, the National Board of Health and Welfare employs assessment results to develop evidence-based guidelines (Glenngard et al., 2005). These are supplied to the government with the overall objective of contributing to the effective use of health-care decisions, within the constructs of health need and an open and transparent priority-setting process. The guidelines include recommendations or decisions on priority-setting and provide national support to assist health-care decision-makers (primarily politicians, civil servants, administrators, providers) in determining effective models of treatment delivery. Specialist associations frequently collaborate in the development of these guidelines and recommendations.

Generally, three versions of each guideline are published – for health-care decision-makers, health-care providers and patients respectively. As directed by the government, the Board must report on the guidelines' projected impact on the practice of medicine (Carlsson, 2004). However, the Board has no direct link with county councils (responsible for regional health-care systems) despite the participation of clinical and economic experts. This may limit the ownership and implementation of guidelines. Since 2006, guidelines have been, or are being, developed for cardiac care, cancer (three most common forms), stroke, venous thrombosis, chronic obstructive pulmonary disease, alcohol and drug abuse, depression and anxiety (Glenngard et al., 2005).

Sweden's decentralized health-care system makes it difficult to ascertain HTA's true impact on decision-making and priority-setting. There is a clear process for the dissemination of results, but it is less clear how such information is used in national and local decision-making. On a national level, there is evidence that certain SBU reports (e.g. stomach pain, smoking cessation) have had an impact on clinical guidance and practice, and facilitated greater support for HTA (Carlsson, 2004). A review of the LFN by Anell & Persson (2005) suggests that health economic evaluation, particularly information on CE, can support decision-making related to reimbursement. However, a minimal percentage of reimbursement decisions to date have been supported by substantial health economic evidence. The majority of LFN decisions have concerned price changes on listed drugs, which normally would not require the support of economic evaluation. Moreover, health economic evidence appears to have the most significant impact on coverage decisions on drugs with broad use (therefore large potential budget impacts) and when CE varies by indication or patient subpopulation. In these cases, the LFN relies more heavily on detailed health economic analyses from manufacturers. It is possible that the LFN will rely increasingly on health economic evidence to support decision-making for reviews of other medicines.

At local level, assessments are used most effectively for decisions on intermediate (e.g. hospitals) and clinical resource allocation and treatment guidelines (Carlsson, 2004). County councils have responsibility for drug expenditures and most local formulary committees lack health economic expertise so, although LFN's decisions influence the recommendations of local formulary committees, local coverage decisions are more restrictive (Anell & Persson, 2005). This results in uncoordinated national and local decision-making.

Other factors influence assessments' impacts on decision-making. These include the time required to complete systematic reviews and evaluate manufacturers' data (in the case of LFN); policy-makers' attitudes to economic information; and complex HTA results that do not always provide a clear policy perspective (Carlsson, 2004). Moreover, HTA has a general problem with limited funds and researchers in small countries like Sweden. While this restricts the ability to address the large number of unevaluated technologies, Sweden strives to ameliorate this by strengthening international collaboration on HTA activities. Specifically, the SBU participates in a number of international endeavours including EUR-ASSESS, HTAi, EuroScan and the International Network of Agencies for Health Technology Assessment (INAHTA, EUnetHTA). In addition, the LFN and SBU collaborate on reviews of groups of drugs. In fact, Sweden is a country with significant collaboration between the HTA and reimbursement agencies.

Table A1.1. *Overview of HTA governance, processes and role in decision-making in Sweden*

Sweden

HTA governance & organization

Institutions/committees	LFN – reimbursement and pricing decisions.
	RFV – pricing decisions.
	SBU – primary national HTA body.
	Ministry of Health and Social Affairs/National Board of Health and Welfare – oversees other institutions; Board issues health-care guidelines.
Entities responsible for reviewing HTA evidence for priority-setting and decision-making	LFN.
	Various health-care decision-makers utilize SBU reports.
HTA agenda-setting body(s)	Predominantly Ministry of Health and Social Affairs; Swedish Parliament.
Areas for HTA	New approved and already reimbursed prescription drugs.
Reimbursement requirements and limitations	Reimbursement depends on yes/no decision for inclusion on positive list. In exceptions, conditional coverage given for particular applications or conditions.
Stakeholder involvement	LFN Board – health economists, medical experts and professionals, representatives of consumer and patient groups.
	SBU – health-care providers, health economists, representatives from health-care organizations.
International collaboration	Secretariat of INAHTA located at the SBU; SBU participates in EuroScan, HTA-related trainings and conferences, EUnetHTA, HTAi and WHO's Health Evidence Network (HEN). SBU also collaborates on multinational projects, most at Nordic and European levels.

HTA topic selection & analytical design

Governance of topic selection	Ministry of Health and Social Affairs, Swedish Parliament, various health-care organizations, health experts and SBU Board.
Criteria for topic selection	SBU: • health impact • breadth of health • societal and ethical considerations • professional or organizational impact • methodological requirements for assessment • technology cost • technology relevance. LFN: Based on manufacturer submission and/or sales volume in each product group.
Criteria for assessment	Therapeutic benefit, patient benefit, CE, availability of therapeutic alternatives, equity considerations.
Criteria outlined or publicly-available	Yes.
Analysis perspective	Societal.
Duration required to conduct assessments	Broad health issues: 3-4 years; single indications or products: shorter period, typically up to 1 year.

Evidence requirements & assessment methods[27]

Documents required from manufacturer	LFN requires summary of up-to-date scientific knowledge including references, clinical and health economics studies (with modelling, if applicable). Manufacturers must present data on actual prescription volumes.

(cont.)

27. Section applies primarily to the LFN.

Table A1.1. *(cont.)*

Systematic literature review and synthesis	Yes.
Unpublished data/ grey literature	Yes.
Preferred clinical study type/ evidence	RCT.
Type of economic assessment preferred or required	Cost-benefit-value analysis, cost-benefit analysis, cost-minimizing analysis with constant health status.
Availability of guidelines outlining methodological requirements	Yes.
Choice of comparator	Requires 3 well-defined comparators for new pharmaceuticals, typically – routine practice, non-medical intervention and do-nothing. For positive list approval, product is compared with all drugs in a therapeutic group – oriented on the second and fourth level of the WHO ATC classification.
Specification of outcome variable	Morbidity, mortality, life quality (QALY) and willingness to pay (WTP). Preference for measures under daily conditions or routine treatment.
Sub-group analyses	For sex, age, disease stage or severity, co-morbidities, risk factors and treatment strategies (e.g. primary/secondary prevention).
Costs included in analysis	Direct and indirect; pharmaceutical costs established on basis of pharmacy costs.
Incremental analyses required	Yes.

Time horizon	Period within which main differences of health effects and costs appear.
Equity issues	Equity considered in decision-making. Analysis does not state how this is accounted for.
Discounting	Costs and benefits: 3% (base analysis), 0%, 3%, 5% and 0%, for costs and benefits respectively (sensitivity analysis).
Modelling	Performed by companies and institutions.
Sensitivity analyses	For central assumptions.
CE or willingness-to-pay threshold	No formal threshold, but likely ranges between £25 000-£40 000 employed.
Missing or incomplete data	Reported problems with poorly presented data from sponsors.
Support for methodological development	Not available.

HTA dissemination & implementation

Channels for dissemination of HTA results	Yellow, White and Alert reports; SBU newsletter; professional conferences, seminars and courses; academic journals; and guidances.
Use of HTA results	Reimbursement, pricing and health-care delivery (via guidelines).
Evidence considered in decision-making	Severity of condition, evidence of effectiveness, CE, price, equity.

(cont.)

Table A1.1. *(cont.)*

Any reported obstacles to effective implementation	Decentralized decision-making structure; policy perspective of HTA results not always clear; attitudes towards economic information in decision-making/priority-setting; time required to complete systematic reviews and evaluate manufacturers' data (in case of LFN).
Formal processes to measure impact	No formal process, but has participated in EUR-ASSESS project that studies HTA's effect on coverage of policy decisions.
Processes for re-evaluation or appeals	Following preliminary decision, sponsors' representatives may present arguments directly to the PPB. Manufacturer can appeal to an independent court if dissatisfied with the final decision.
Accountability for stakeholder input	Stakeholders that subscribe to SBU Alert reports may comment following publication on the Internet.
Transparent/public decision-making process	LFN: Board's decisions are outlined in a document available on its web site. Includes arguments for each decision.

Sources: Anell & Persson, 2005; Zentner et al., 2005; Carlsson, 2004; OECD, 2003; International Society for Pharmacoeconomics and Outcomes Research (ISPOR), 1999.

Appendix 2. The Netherlands

Overview of health-care and reimbursement systems

Under the Constitution, every Dutch citizen in the Netherlands is entitled to health care founded on social insurance principles. This health-care system is characterized by a complex array of institutions, regulations and responsibilities (Bos, 2000). Public health care, infectious disease control, environmental protection and the regulation of health-care professionals form an integral part of central government, particularly the Ministry of Health, Welfare and Sport (den Exter et al., 2004). Service delivery typically rests with independent practitioners or non-profit service organizations (Stolk & Rutten, 2005; Bos, 2000). Consequently, health care in the Netherlands consists of an interdependent mix of public and private initiatives under the umbrella of central government. On a macro-level, this translates to collaborative and interrelated policy processes and decision-making across public, private and professional stakeholders.

The public-private interplay of responsibility and decision-making power extends to the financing of health care. The Sickness Fund Act (1996) implemented a compulsory national health insurance scheme in the Netherlands (den Exter et al., 2004). Originally the sickness fund covered about 63% of the population through the social security system; others were insured through a similar social insurance scheme (for employees of provincial and municipal governmental bodies) or private plans (den Exter et al., 2004). Since January 2006, statutory and private health insurance have been integrated within one comprehensive package – the basisverzekering (basic health-care insurance policy). This covers the entire population under national health insurance and includes all acute care provided by hospitals, general practitioners and specialists; all drug and appliance costs; and transportation. As of 2004, there were 22 sickness funds, all overseen by the Health Care Insurance Board (CVZ) (den Exter et al., 2004). This represents the government, employers, employees, insurance funds, health-care institutions and health professionals.

The Ministry of Health, Welfare and Sport implements the Dutch Government's pharmaceutical policy, guided by the principle of safe and affordable pharmaceutical care for all. The Medicines Evaluation Board (MEB), under the auspices of the MEB Agency, evaluates and regulates access to the market as the quality and appropriate use of pharmaceuticals is integral to public health protection. Specifically, new pharmaceuticals are registered following evidence of quality, safety and efficacy (Stolk & Rutten, 2005). Historically, this registration resulted in practically automatic reimbursement by health insurance bodies (den Exter et al., 2004). However, in attempts to control costs and assure equitable access to pharmaceutical care, the Ministry increasingly has required evidence of CE prior to admission in the benefits package (positive list) covered by the sickness funds. Conversely, the Government can remove ineffective or obsolete pharmaceuticals from the package[28] and, under the Pharmaceutical Pricing Act 1996, sets the prices of pharmaceutical products.

As indicated, not all registered drugs qualify for reimbursement. In particular, pharmaceuticals are reimbursed by the sickness fund only if they are admitted to either of the schedules in the positive list. Schedule A includes a reference price system[29] with groups of substitutive pharmaceuticals; Schedule B lists drugs with alternatives (Fig. A2.1).

Pharmaceuticals are included in Schedule A if they are substitutes for existing drugs. In the Netherlands, it is mandated that medicines be merged in one group (a cluster) if they address similar indications and a comparable method of administration, with no clinically relevant differences in their properties (Stolk & Rutten, 2005). It is assumed that at least one medicine in each group is fully reimbursable.

If a new pharmaceutical has no available appropriate and mutually replaceable substitute (therefore the reference price system does not apply), the manufacturer can apply for an evaluation from the Ministry of Health, Welfare and Sport[30] (Zentner et al., 2005; den Exter et al., 2004). The assessment is conducted by the Pharmaceutical Care Committee (CFH), the body responsible for valuing pharmaceuticals and providing the Ministry with recommendations for the positive list (see the following section HTA process and procedures). Following a CFH recommendation, supported by the Ministry, the pharmaceutical is included in Schedule B for reimbursement.[31] Reimbursement conditions for the positive list are uniform for both public and private payers (Stolk & Rutten, 2005). While the majority of products are reimbursed fully, limits can

---

28. In 1996, pharmaceuticals in the health benefits package were evaluated on the basis of need and effectiveness, in order to streamline and improve the quality of the overall package. The process resulted in the removal of a significant number of pharmaceuticals (as of April 1996).

29. The level of reimbursement is based on the average price of pharmaceuticals in a comparable group.

30. Manufacturers must explain for which part of the positive list the proposed pharmaceutical seems to be qualified.

31. Since 1999, new drugs with higher prices than existing substitutes may be reimbursed if efficacy and effectiveness requirements are satisfied. Moreover, since 2005, a pharmacoeconomic study and budget impact analysis is formally required for a new drug with a premium price.

Fig. A2.1 *Reimbursement decision process in the Netherlands.*

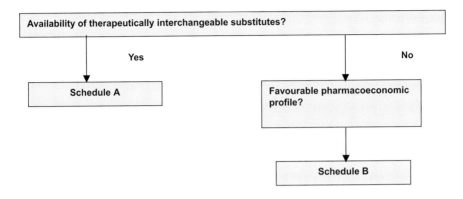

Source: Stolk & Rutten, 2005.

be set. For example, reimbursement may be restricted to a particular patient population or for use by a certain medical specialty.

The CFH is part of the CVZ and comprises 18 members, representing pharmacists, specialist physicians, economists, psychologists, epidemiologists and ministry representatives (Zentner et al., 2005). External medical experts support the assessment process according to the particular assessment.

HTA governance and organization

The use and visibility of HTA in the Netherlands has grown over the last 20 years. This is primarily a result of expansions in health technology, growth in health-care costs and a subsequent increase in the regulation of medical products (den Exter et al., 2004). In particular, throughout the 1980s, politicians and policy-makers increased the pressure for systematic evaluation of new medical technology to support decision-making and improve health-care status and provision. The Health Insurance Council[32] required all new technological innovations to undergo CE analysis prior to determination of coverage in the benefit package (Berg et al., 2004). Moreover, there was a push to institutionalize HTA and improve coordination of assessment activities throughout the Netherlands.

Three influential advisory bodies – the Health Insurance Council, the Health Council of the Netherlands and the National Council for Public

---

32. Now the Health Care Insurance Board.

Health – established a National Fund for Investigative Medicine[33] in 1998 (den Exter et al., 2004). Administered by the Dutch Health Research and Development Council (formerly overseen by the Health Insurance Council), the fund's primary aim was to finance original research in support of scientific excellence and evidence-based policy-making (Berg et al., 2004; Bos, 2000). This included the evaluation of new and existing medical technologies, including the associated CE and social, ethical and regulatory implications for the particular policy question or decision required (Bos, 2000). In essence, this served as the national HTA programme, supported primarily by the Ministry of Health, Welfare and Sport and of Education, Culture and Science (Berg et al., 2004). Recently the fund was replaced by the Netherlands Organisation for Health Research and Development (ZonMw), a merger of the Netherlands Organization for Scientific Research (NWO) and the existing Netherlands Organisation for Health Research and Development (ZON) (see below).

Several pivotal reports on streamlining the benefits package and improving the appropriate use of medical products were released following this merger. These further established HTA's role in the health-care system (Berg et al., 2004; den Exter et al., 2004). More recently, the Dutch Parliament has become increasingly interested in HTA and has requested status reports on these activities from the Minister of Health (Banta, 2003).

The Health Council of the Netherlands is one of the primary institutions for economic evaluation. It is funded entirely by the Dutch Government, with budget contributions from various relevant ministries. Established in 1902, this is an independent statutory body that advises the government (ministers and parliament) on medicine, health care, public health and environmental issues (Berg et al., 2004). Standing and ad-hoc committees report on specific topics requested (Health Council of the Netherlands, 2006). Committees comprise council members and external experts (approximately 200) from various medical specialties and scientific disciplines. Typically, these committees evaluate the effectiveness, efficiency, safety and availability of health interventions. Some committees may also examine specific epidemiological and economic aspects, as well as associated ethical, social and legal issues. There are approximately 40 to 50 committees at any given time, each with an average of 10 experts (Health Council of the Netherlands, 2006). The composition of each committee reflects the need for both appropriate scientific expertise and a multidisciplinary perspective.

---

33. Before the Fund was established, the three Councils advised the Dutch government that HTA should be viewed and utilized as an important aid to decision-making. The Health Council delineated an ideal HTA system and how this could improve the effectiveness of policy decisions.

The Health Council also serves an alerting function by providing unsolicited advice on various topics and related ministerial policy. Interests and activities range from health prevention and treatment (e.g. cochlear implants for children, bioterrorism, immunization) to nutrition and the environment (e.g. radiation). Work specific to HTA was undertaken during the late 1990s and early 2000s (primarily via an interim Central Committee on Medical Technology Assessment), but such activities were reduced significantly in 2003 due to lack of funding (Health Council of the Netherlands, 2005). However, in mid-2005, the Council published a report recommending that projects specific to HTA be increased and supported.

Several other organizations involved in HTA activities in the Netherlands are detailed below (Berg et al., 2004; den Exter et al., 2004; Bos, 2000).

- *Netherlands Organisation for Health Research and Development (ZonMw).* National health council appointed by the Ministry of Health and the NWO to promote quality and innovation in health research and care. Responsible for the programming, priority-setting and allocation of government funds for research projects in health care and prevention. In particular, the ZonMw Health Care Efficiency Research programme has an annual budget of €12.2 million to actively support CE studies and implementation research. The programme focuses on services covered by health insurance including diagnostics; therapy and care; and organizations in all medical and paramedical disciplines.

- *Netherlands Organization for Scientific Research (NWO).* A statutory organization with the primary goal of improving the quality of health-related research in the Netherlands. Acts as a national general research council, playing a significant role in the development of science, technology and culture, including the medical sector. Has supported several HTA initiatives and projects over the last 20 years.

- *Council for Public Health and Health Care (RVZ).* Instituted in 1995 as an independent body that advises the government on public health and care. Primarily issues advisory reports on government health-care policy covering prevention, health protection, general health care and care of the elderly and people with disabilities. Moreover, reports cover various policy aspects including insurance, planning, financing, training and patient rights.

- *National Institute for Public Health and the Environment (RIVM).* Engages in a number of activities related to technology assessment, with the main task of evaluating and monitoring vaccines. Also evaluates certain medical devices, particularly those requiring sterilization.

- *Netherlands Institute of Primary Health Care.* Independent, non-profit research body with broad expertise in health-service research including technology assessment on topics such as quality systems, home-care technologies and the evaluation of professional procedures. Board of Governors comprises health-care providers, health insurers, patients/consumers and academics.

- *Netherlands Organization for Applied Scientific Research (TNO).* Foremost biomedical technology institute in the Netherlands. Limited assessment activity, but evaluates medical devices and is actively involved in coordinating EU-wide HTA projects (Bos, 2000). Evaluation activities focus on policy aspects of technology development and diffusion, home-care technology and minimally invasive therapies. Established programme on preventive medicine has issued various HTA reports.

- *Dutch Institute for Healthcare Improvement (CBO).* Active in quality assurance and technology assessment. Plays significant role in consensus and guideline development.

- *Various academic institutes.* Erasmus University Rotterdam plays the most prominent role in HTA in the Dutch academic community. The Institute for Medical Technology Assessment (iMTA) is the largest group dedicated to HTA. Its primary focus is economic evaluation of health technologies, as well as quality assessment of health care. Many projects are carried out in collaboration with health-care providers, particularly hospitals, affiliated with the Fund for Investigative Medicine. The Department of Public Health and the Centre for Health Policy and Law are also involved in HTA-related activities.

Beyond Erasmus University, the Department of Health Economics at the University of Limburg is involved in HTA activities, indeed virtually all medical faculties and university hospitals in the Netherlands have some involvement in HTA endeavours.

While the organizations listed provide much of the driving force, several smaller organizations undertake HTA activities. Consequently, HTA in the Netherlands is neither concentrated on, nor directed by, one national research and policy organization. Unlike in other EU countries (e.g. Sweden) many different entities, with often divergent research agendas and traditions, must come together to support national policy and priority-setting activities. Despite greater coordination and improved integration between entities historically organized around the Fund for Investigative Medicine, better cooperation and harmonization is needed.

HTA process and procedures

Although HTA has adequate resources they are not sufficient to evaluate all new and existing health technologies. This has resulted in an increased focus on setting priorities in order to exploit HTA's potential to improve the efficiency and quality of health care in the Netherlands.

In the early days of the Fund, most assessments focused on new, high-cost, sophisticated therapies, with minimal concern for existing technologies (Bos, 2000). The submission, selection and funding of projects often lacked direct links to health-care areas of greatest concern or most underdeveloped. Also, few evaluations examined the social, ethical and legal implications of health technology (den Exter et al., 2004). These problems caused a significant disconnect between most HTA research and heath-care need, policy development and decision-making. Concern over these prioritizing methods led to efforts to make the process more explicit and rational, and to incorporate social and scientific criteria to determine HTA priorities (Berg et al., 2004).

Throughout the 1990s, the primary actors in the identification and setting of HTA priorities (e.g. CVZ, Health Council, Council for Medical and Health Research – (ZonMw) undertook formal processes to identify technologies or areas of health care requiring assessment[34] (Oortwijin et al., 2002). The technologies were ranked according to a range of criteria: degree of uncertainty concerning efficacy and effectiveness; frequency of use; costs; impact on morbidity, mortality and quality of life; and rate of use (Berg et al., 2004). Priority topics for evaluation included ultrasound therapy, treatment for urinary incontinence, long-term psychotherapy and diagnostic testing.

Currently, research proposals are submitted to the CVZ for evaluation and reviewed by members of the Committee for Investigative Medicine and the Board. Specifically, the reviews independently evaluate, rate and score the policy relevance of the submitted proposals based on a variety of objective criteria[35] (Oortwijin et al., 2002):

- actual burden of disease, given current treatment strategies for the individual patient;

- potential benefit for the individual patient;

---

34. Typical formal process – expert consultation and topic nomination; prioritization via Delphi-based process; further ranking; creation of nominated HTA-subject lists.

35. Researchers submitting proposals are explicitly requested to provide information about the policy relevance of the proposed project. Moreover, reviewers apply a standardized weighting system to the selection criteria to rate and score each proposal.

- number of patients;

- intervention's direct costs per patient;

- financial consequences of applying the intervention over time (impact on total costs of health care);

- additional aspects with impacts on health policy (e.g. potential rate of diffusion).

Proposals considered to have intermediate to high policy relevance are sent to the CMHR (Oortwijn et al., 2002). These are appraised for scientific quality and accepted, declined or recommended for revision before resubmission. The Health Council of the Netherlands prioritizes assessments according to requests from ministries and parliament and of its own volition. Topics for further assessment and funding are generated directly by the Ministry or via input from expert working groups that formulate funding programmes. The various priority lists described above also help to shape these agendas.

In addition to the publication of advisory reports requested by government, the Health Council's remit includes horizon-scanning. This draws attention proactively to health issues and developments that may be relevant to government policy and associated agenda-setting (Health Council of the Netherlands, 2005). The Health Council's primary scanning activities focus on preventive and curative health care; nutrition and food quality; environment and health; and work and health. Its secretariat participates in EuroScan to identify significant emerging health technologies for preventive and curative health care. Horizon-scanning also involves the identification of ethical and legal aspects of public health-related scientific developments that may have policy implications.

Various assessment and research organizations in the Netherlands complete numerous HTA assessments and research each year, based primarily on extensive literature review (e.g. systematic literature review, meta-analysis) and consultation with expert groups (Bos, 2000). In general, the Health Council and CVZ publish some 20 to 30 reports annually. The range of assessments is quite expansive, as illustrated below (Health Council of the Netherlands, 2005; Bos, 2000).

- use of biosynthetic human growth hormone treatment (*CVZ*);

- use of lung transplantation (*CVZ*);

- use of diagnostic imaging techniques for back pain (*CVZ*);

- extra-corporeal membrane oxygenation treatment in neonates (*Health Council*);

- cholesterol-lowering therapy (*Health Council*);

- silicone breast implants (*Health Council*);

- nanotechnologies (*Health Council*); and

- use of antiviral agents and other measures in an influenza pandemic (*Health Council*).

As described, the CFH allows reimbursement for new drugs that cannot be substituted, but only if efficiency and effectiveness requirements are met. Manufacturers provide evidence to support the valuation process, including systematic literature reviews or meta-analyses, clinical studies and pharmacoeconomic evaluations (with modelling, if appropriate); consensus guidelines and prescription data (Zentner et al., 2005). In addition, manufacturers typically choose the comparator in accordance with pharmacoeconomic guidelines and may discuss the selection a priori with the relevant assessment body (see Table A2.1). The CFH assesses new medications by comparison with the relevant positive list on a range of criteria, including (Zentner et al., 2005):

- therapeutic value

- patient benefit

- CE

- financial impact on benefits package, pharmaceutical and health budgets, Sickness Fund and Dutch society.

Therapeutic value and patient benefit is determined by comparison with standard or usual therapies. The CFH employs several legally regulated criteria to evaluate the relative therapeutic benefits, particularly efficacy, effectiveness and potential use of a product. Product use is categorized by three classifications (measured by number of prescriptions over time) (Zentner et al., 2005): satisfactory, broad and limited. Satisfactory or broad use are preferred but limited application does not necessarily result in a negative valuation, especially in cases where the comparator is more expensive. Other relevant criteria include the availability of therapeutic alternatives; disease severity; target patient population; the mode, frequency and comfort of drug delivery; and impact on the quality of life (Zentner et al., 2005). All criteria are important but efficacy, effectiveness and the side-effect profile carry greater weight. Whether the product is a breakthrough therapy or the only available treatment for a condition(s) are critical factors in determining additional therapeutic benefit (Zentner et al., 2005). Other criteria, such as affordability and leakage (use of a product outside the designated patient group) are also considered , albeit less often, in reimbursement decisions (Stolk & Rutten, 2005).

Having assessed clinical value, the CFH requires economic evaluations (e.g. CE or cost-benefit analysis) of pharmaceuticals for which manufacturers claim therapeutic benefits. Moreover, since 2005, new drugs with a price premium have been required to undergo economic studies and budget-impact analyses (Stolk & Rutten, 2005). These must be carried out and submitted by manufacturers. In 1999, the Health Insurance Board issued pharmacoeconomic guidelines to standardize this research across the Netherlands and, particularly, manufacturers' applications for inclusion in the benefits package (Zentner et al., 2005).

Two pharmaceutical categories are exempt from the standard valuation process, as previously described. The Ministry of Health, Welfare and Sport has decreed that orphan drugs (treatments for conditions of low prevalence, typically <5 per 10 000) do not have to undergo economic evaluation (European Commission, 2006). In addition, there is an expedited appraisal process for drugs that treat life-threatening illnesses (i.e. therapeutic breakthrough), and those that are the only available therapy for a given condition.

Following an appraisal, the CFH sets out its recommendations in an assessment report that is published on the Internet and submitted to the Minister of Health. CFH recommendations supported by the Ministry are included in the second section (Schedule B) of the positive list.

HTA dissemination and implementation

In general, activities that employ the results of assessments have the following applications (Bos, 2000):

- address knowledge gaps on innovative technologies and disseminates this knowledge to relevant stakeholder groups;
- decide on the coverage or reimbursement of technologies in the benefit package (in the case of the CFH);
- define or redefines a technology's established indications in order to promote appropriate use;
- establish guidelines for use in order to reduce significant and/or unexplained practice variations; and
- underpin planning and regulation for priority-setting or estimating the future need for a health technology.

Economic assessments submitted to, and reviewed by, the CFH are used for reimbursement and pricing decisions; the Health Council uses HTA predominantly for priority-setting and the production of guidelines. Health Council reports are presented to the Minister of Health who assumes responsibility for their implementation. To facilitate the process, all reports contain recommendations or guidance for implementing the results (Bos, 2000). Several reports have resulted in the development of practice guidelines. For example, the effectiveness and appropriateness of auxiliary tests (e.g. X-ray, ECG) were established through assessment that formed the basis for new practice guidelines on preoperative routine screening (Bos, 2000).

The Health Council not only provides reports directly to the Minister, but also disseminates assessment results through a variety of channels. The Council publishes a bi-monthly Dutch-language journal – *Graadmeter* – containing information about advisory reports and other publications, as well as questions and responses from ministers and state secretaries (Health Council of the Netherlands, 2005). The journal also features brief articles on national and international developments with direct relevance to the Council's fields of interest. The Council distributes *Network* three times a year to international contacts and colleagues. This provides information on the Council's activities and potential opportunities for collaboration. Information also is disseminated via a web site (where many reports are publicly available in both Dutch and English) and conferences.

International collaboration is a key mechanism for strengthening the scientific rigour and implementation of assessments. Frequently, the Council recruits international experts to participate on assessment committees, and exchanges reports with similar organizations abroad. It is a member of EuroScan and other European-based organizations and often collaborates with the Institute of Medicine (IOM) and Centers for Disease Control and Prevention (CDC) in the United States.

The CVZ also disseminates reports (primarily directly to the Minister of Health) that are intended to support reimbursement decisions. The majority focus on diagnostic and therapeutic procedures and the Ministry has implemented a number of these recommendations. The effectiveness and CE of lung transplantation was established via economic assessment and subsequently approved for inclusion in the benefit package (Bos, 2000).

While HTA results are integral to the development of practice guidelines, the two are only beginning to converge in the Netherlands. The chief and established guideline development programmes (the CBO and the Dutch College of General Practitioners – NHG) draw upon evidence found in the literature and, increasingly, completed technology assessments (Berg et al., 2004). Typically, they select guidelines topics based on expert consensus meetings which are also used to refine the development process. Recently the CBO and NHG have begun to coordinate activities and steer towards similar methodologies (Berg et al., 2004).

As in the HTA process, guideline development rarely incorporates normative considerations systematically, such as the patient's perspective in the health-care decision-making process (Berg et al., 2004). While patients have a role in clinical studies, this is more limited in priority-setting, substantiating recommendations and implementing results in the Netherlands (as in most countries). Patient and consumer involvement in decision-making has been strengthened by representation from entities such as the Federation of Patients and Consumer Organisations. This represents patient and consumer interests on national advisory bodies such as the CVZ and the National Council for Health Care (Bos, 2000). That said, there is limited consumer participation in determining the direction of health policy, including HTA. This tends to be influenced significantly by scientific advisory bodies, special committees and medical societies in the Netherlands.

While HTA has certainly generated overall greater awareness of the importance and relevance of economic information in decision-making in the Netherlands, its impact upon the overall policy and priority-setting process remains limited. This narrow application may be due, in part, to the topic selection process and relative lack of coordination between the many different agencies that prioritize, fund and execute HTA research, and to the unequal application of HTA results and decisions implemented by government (Berg et al., 2004).

Sometimes HTA analyses are performed explicitly to guide national policy and, increasingly, support decision-making processes. Yet, some decisions go against available HTA evidence – often technologies are introduced without any economic evaluation and the list of excluded services is still minimal and highly diverse (Berg et al., 2004). A recent Council for Public Health and Health Care report (2006) emphasizes the need for more systematic application of HTA criteria and evidence in decision-making. In particular, the Council argues that, thus far:

> ...decisions regarding payment or non-payment for medical treatment are only based to a limited degree on 'hard' factors, such as CE, and much more on less transparent considerations, as a result of pressure by lobby groups, media, etc. This means that limits [to reimbursement] are indeed being set at present, but on an ad hoc and somewhat random basis. The result is that the available resources are not being deployed as efficiently as possible.

The Council goes on to promulgate a system of decision-making that is transparent and sustainable, based on the "justifiable" and "coherent" application of criteria for establishing priorities for the public financing of health care. By "justifiable", the Council suggests that criteria should be fair and equitable from the perspective of the general public and their use should guarantee equal access to health care. A "coherent" use of criteria employs a model with distinct assessment and appraisal phases. The assessment phase covers quantitative evaluation of an invention, based on necessity, effectiveness and CE. The appraisal phase involves the consideration of social aspects and other non-quantifiable factors. The Council highlights that "… should the outcome of the societal examination be different from that of the assessment phase, the new verdict should be explicitly justified." Moreover, it suggests the use of an explicit maximum CE threshold (around €80 000 per QALY gained) to function as a decision rule to maximize transparent decision-making.

Having made effective use of HTA evidence in decision-making, the impact of resulting actions (e.g. guideline development) may be hampered by lack of resources, knowledge and incentives for policy-makers and providers to utilize the information in actual decision-making and treatment provision.

Table A2.1. *Overview of HTA governance, processes and role in decision-making in the Netherlands*

The Netherlands

HTA governance & organization

Institutions/committees	CFH – reimbursement and pricing negotiations. ZonMw Many smaller organizations and entities (described above).
Entities responsible for reviewing HTA evidence for priority-setting and decision-making	CVZ; CFH; Ministry of Health, Welfare and Sport.
HTA agenda-setting body(s)	Primarily, Ministry of Health, Welfare and Sport; CVZ, CMHR; and Health Council. Other organizations such as the ZonMW and the NWO also fund HTA activities and set priorities for research.
Areas for HTA	New, approved and already reimbursed prescription drugs (CFH); variety of health-care interventions (Health Council).

(cont.)

Table A2.1. *(cont.)*

Reimbursement requirements and limitations	Reimbursement depends on yes/no decision for admission to reference pricing system. In exceptions, conditional coverage given for particular applications or conditions.
Stakeholder involvement	Medical and health-care professionals and experts, insurance funds and representatives from consumer associations (Health Council, CMHR, CVZ). Limited patient and public involvement in HTA process.
International collaboration	EuroScan, AGREE Collaboration, EUnetHTA, IOM, CDC, INAHTA (Health Council, CVZ).

HTA topic selection & analytical design

Governance of topic selection	CHF: based on manufacturers' submissions. Other: CVZ; Health Council; Ministry of Health, Welfare and Sport.
Criteria for topic selection	• burden of disease • potential benefit for individual patients • number of patients • cost of technology i.e. cost per patient and total costs • additional aspects related to health policy. Health Council also selects topics for horizon-scanning based on relevance to government policy and associated agenda-setting.
Criteria for assessment	Therapeutic benefit, patient benefit, CE, budget impact, pharmaceutical/innovative characteristics and availability of therapeutic alternatives. Other social, ethical and legal considerations, as appropriate.
Criteria outlined or publicly-available	Yes.
Analysis perspective	Societal.

Duration required to conduct assessments	From few months to one year or more.

Evidence requirements & assessment methods[36]

Documents required from manufacturer	Systematic literature review or meta-analyses, clinical studies and pharmacoeconomic evaluations (with modelling, if appropriate), consensus guidelines and prescription data.
Systematic literature review and synthesis	Yes.
Unpublished data/ grey literature	Yes.
Preferred clinical study type/ evidence	Blind head-to-head RCTs.
Type of economic assessment preferred or required	CE and cost-utility analysis.
Availability of guidelines outlining methodological requirements	Provided by CVZ.
Choice of comparator	Standard therapy (routine daily practice) or common therapy. Pharmaceuticals must be compared against listed drugs.
Specification of outcome variable	Mortality, morbidity, QALY, costs.
Sub-group analyses	Amongst other patient groups, extent of disease and severity, co-morbidity. A priori definitions must be established.

(cont.)

---

36. Section primarily refers to the CFH.

Table A2.1. *(cont.)*

Costs included in analysis	Direct costs both inside and outside the health-care system. Future health-care costs for unrelated disease in any additional life should be excluded. Productivity losses calculated using the friction cost method should be presented separately.
Incremental analyses required	Yes.
Time horizon	Period within which main differences of health effects and costs appear.
Equity issues	Social perspective preferred.
Discounting	Costs (4%), benefits (1.5%).
Modelling	Performed by manufacturers.
Sensitivity analyses	Performed on central assumptions; employ univariate and multivariate analysis methods.
CE or willingness-to-pay threshold	No formal threshold. Use of an explicit threshold is currently being promulgated and discussed, with potential for different thresholds according to severity of disease.
Missing or incomplete data	Not available.
Support for methodological development	Not available.

HTA dissemination & implementation

Channels for HTA results dissemination	CFH: decisions/recommendations outlined in assessment report published on the Internet and delivered to relevant ministries.
	Health Council: Graadmeter, Network, web site, international conferences and collaboration with related agencies (national and international)

Use of HTA results	Reimbursement and pricing decisions; provide relevant stakeholders with information on health technologies' effectiveness and CE ; inform appropriate clinical practice via guidelines; define or redefine established indications for a technology; support priority-setting for government policies.
Evidence considered in decision-making	Efficacy, safety, effectiveness, CE, financial impact, quality of life and social/ethical/legal considerations (where applicable).
Any reported obstacles to effective implementation	Disconnect between policy question, clinical/ practice needs and HTA evidence; lack of coordination between myriad agencies involved in priority-setting, funding and execution of HTA and related activities; health professionals and hospital administrators reluctant to use HTA information; gulf between scientific/technical nature of HTA and subjective/normative environment of health policy-making; guideline development tends to rely on efficacy/ effectiveness data, not CE evidence.
Formal processes to measure impact	No.
Processes for re-evaluation or appeals	Not available.
Accountability for stakeholder input	Not available.
Transparent/public decision-making process	Not available.

Sources: Health Council of the Netherlands, 2006; Stolk & Poley, 2005; Zentner et al., 2005; Berg et al., 2004; den Exter et al., 2004; OECD, 2003; Bos, 2000; ISPOR, 1999.

Appendix 3. Finland

Overview of health-care and reimbursement systems

Finland has a long tradition of supporting social programmes that promote equity and the welfare state. For example, universal access to medical care is guaranteed for all residents and provided by public health centres and hospitals. Moreover, health policy and planning tends to be based on a holistic approach that encompasses prevention and health promotion, community involvement, multi-sectoral collaboration and international cooperation.

Organization and financing of health care in Finland have long been considered to be public responsibilities. Each of the country's five provinces is run by a provincial government that monitors the provision of health care (Lauslahti et al., 2000). However, local municipalities arrange and provide care for their citizens (Jarvelin, 2002).[37] Since 2005, there are 432 municipalities with between 1000 and 500 000 inhabitants. The main basic services provided by local authorities are prescribed by law but the scope, content and organization of services differ between municipalities.

At the national level, the Ministry of Social Affairs and Health directs and guides social and health services. Its remit is to define general policy; prepare major reforms and proposals for legislation and monitor implementation; and assist the government in decision-making (Jarvelin, 2002). In addition, the Ministry finances health-care policy research in collaboration with the Social Insurance Institution (Kela), the Academy of Finland, universities and private foundations.

Several agencies and institutions affiliated to the Ministry are responsible for various areas of health care (Jarvelin, 2002; Lauslahti et al., 2000).

- *National Research and Development Centre for Welfare and Health (STAKES).* Monitors and evaluates activities in health-care services and carries out R&D.

- *National Authority for Medicolegal Affairs.* Regulates health professionals and the legal protection of patients.

- *National Agency for Medicines (NAM).* Maintains and promotes safe use of medicines, medical devices and blood products. Performs preliminary

---

37. The 1972 Primary Health Care Act requires municipalities to provide health promotion and disease prevention, medical care, medical rehabilitation and dental care. It also mandates the provision of student and occupational health care, screening services, family planning services, mental health care and ambulance services.

examination of applications for marketing authorization and monitors manufacture, importation and distribution of medicines.

- *National Public Health Institute.* Carries out research on diseases and their prevention. Also undertakes surveillance and survey activities on communicable diseases and health behaviour.

Central government and local authorities form the main levels of health-care organization, but the private sector also plays a role. Private health care comprises mainly outpatient care, predominantly in larger urban areas, provided via a physiotherapy unit or medical care practice (Jarvelin, 2002).

The health-care system in Finland is primarily tax-based. Most financing is derived from municipal taxes levied (almost 50%) for health services (Jarvelin, 2002). Local authorities also receive state subsidies to arrange health care, social programmes and education. Other financing comes from the state, the National Health Insurance (NHI) scheme and private sources (e.g. households).

The NHI scheme is overseen by Kela (under the auspices of parliament). This covers loss of income during illness, pharmaceuticals, private and occupational health care and some other services (Jarvelin, 2002). The proportion of health care financed by the NHI has increased as pharmaceutical costs grew significantly during the 1990s in Finland, mainly because of the growing use of new drugs. Cost containment has been addressed by a number of actions initiated over the last 10 years. One measure requires the therapeutic value and CE of new drugs to be demonstrated before granting eligibility for reimbursement.[38]

Under the auspices of the Ministry of Social Affairs and Health, the Pharmaceuticals Pricing Board (PPB) is responsible for evaluating, pricing and approving reimbursements of new pharmaceuticals, patented drugs and generics. Before a drug can be licensed as reimbursable its wholesale price determined by the PPB must be deemed reasonable (Zentner et al., 2005). The reasonable wholesale price refers to the maximum price at which a drug may be sold to pharmacies and hospitals (Jarvelin, 2002). The PPB also deals with applications to increase the wholesale prices of medicines.

The PPB comprises seven representatives appointed by the Ministry: two members from the Ministry of Social Affairs and Health, Ministry of Finance and Kela respectively and at least one medical, pharmacology, economic or legal expert.

---

38. Finland has three reimbursement tiers with corresponding co-payment categories. The basic tier has a subgroup for "significant and "expensive" drugs, with 50% reimbursement. The second and third categories cover drugs that treat chronic conditions and those required to maintain health status or normal bodily functions. Reimbursements for these categories range from 75% to 100% and are publicly financed.

HTA governance and organization

In the early 1990s, the Academy of Finland and the National Board of Health released separate reports emphasizing the need for assessment of medical technologies and the establishment of research entities to conduct such activities (Jarvelin, 2002). Several organizations, such as universities and hospitals, were active in HTA during the 1980s, but there was little cooperation and collaboration. The National Board of Health proposed the establishment of a national technology unit at the Ministry of Social Affairs and Health and identified the need for a team of national experts on health technology representing different health-care sectors (Lauslahti et al., 2000). The Finnish Office of Health Technology Assessment (FinOHTA), an independent centre for HTA, was established within STAKES in 1995.

FinOHTA is the central body for the advancement of HTA-related work in Finland, acting as the clearing house for accumulating, evaluating and disseminating knowledge on HTA and evidence-based assessment methods. It supports, coordinates and conducts assessments, and disseminates national and international research results within the health-care system (FinOHTA, 2006). It also monitors the conduct of HTA research, within Finland and abroad, and the development of new research and methods, and prioritizes health technologies in need of assessment. Ultimately, FinOHTA strives to improve the effectiveness and efficiency of Finnish health care.

At present, FinOHTA employs around 13 individuals who provide medical, nursing and economic expertise. In addition, it makes extensive use of an external network of experts in medicine and health care. An advisory board and scientific committee oversee direction and activities (FinOHTA, 2006a; Lauslahti et al., 2000). The advisory board monitors assessment activities within FinOHTA and externally and develops proposals for national and international joint assessment projects. It consists of 26 members representing academic institutions, hospitals, related national health-care institutes, medical societies, consumer groups and medical technology associations. The 13-member scientific committee comprises leading members of Finland's medical-scientific community. It examines priorities in HTA and evaluates the quality and priority of proposed assessment projects. The committee also participates in disseminating HTA information and results.

Within STAKES, FinOHTA has access to health and social services research and resources, international contacts and logistical support (Lauslahti et al., 2000). Moreover, STAKES houses the Norwegian branch of the Nordic Cochrane Centre and maintains official health and social services statistics, registries and databases. FinOHTA also collaborates with other national organizations and bodies, including hospital districts, Duodecim (the Finnish Medical Society), National Public Health Institute and NAM.

FinOHTA also relies heavily on international collaboration. It has initiated joint HTA projects with the SBU and other Nordic assessment bodies (Lauslahti et al., 2000). FinOHTA also participates in INAHTA, EUnetHTA, AGREE collaboration (network to improve clinical practice guidelines) and the Guidelines International Network (G-I-N).

HTA process and procedures

The Ministry of Social Affairs and Health requires assessment activities to concentrate on technologies important for the health of Finnish citizens or the national economy (Lauslahti et al., 2000). FinOHTA is a relatively small organization, with limited staff and funding, so areas of HTA are prioritized by a formalized process for selecting assessment topics and commissioning studies (preliminary studies or comprehensive assessments) from outside organizations and research groups. Priority is given to projects that examine the effectiveness and CE of health-care technologies, as well as systematic literature reviews. The proposed assessment can be part of a larger study or a stand-alone research project.

FinOHTA staff and external consultants review all project submissions, typically every two to three weeks. Project proposals are evaluated against the following criteria (FinOHTA, 2006a):

- impact on public health or national economy;
- appropriateness and quality of proposed research methods;
- feasibility of study;
- adequacy of study aims in assessing effectiveness, CE and other considerations including social, ethical, legal and quality of life implications;
- researcher(s) conflict of interest;
- qualifications of research group or organization;
- appropriate funding structure;
- timely duration required for study completion;
- usability of study results;
- sufficient plan for results' dissemination, implementation and follow-up.

Projects that meet these criteria are presented to the Scientific Committee every two to three months. Approval is granted to those that address suitable topics and possess scientifically valid study designs. A final decision is made when approved projects are presented to STAKES' Board of Directors. The review and decision process typically takes between two and six months.

FinOHTA also conducts a variety of evaluative research, particularly systematic reviews of available evidence. This entails collection, analysis and synthesis of information on a range of economic evaluations that may include national and international assessments and research examining the diffusion of technology and identification of emerging therapies (FinOHTA, 2006a; Lauslahti et al., 2000). Rapid Reviews are one example: FinOHTA produces information on a given health technology that is needed quickly so a comprehensive assessment is not feasible. These reviews typically are based on international assessment reports and the findings are reviewed, appraised and applied to the Finnish context. During systematic review of the available evidence, FinOHTA considers a wide range of assessment factors for the given health technology including therapeutic, patient and cost benefits; CE; quality of life; organizational and service requirements (e.g. need for technologists or staff training); budget impacts; and social, legal and ethical implications (Eskola et al., 2004).

In addition to systematic reviews, FinOHTA utilizes different assessment methodologies according to the particular research question. Such methodological approaches include primary studies (e.g. RCTs) that study the effectiveness and CE of various health technologies (especially when lack of available evidence); surveys to clarify the use of a technology or variations in practice; and modelling (e.g. costs associated with different approaches to technology utilization) (Eskola et al., 2004).

Clinicians are involved frequently in the assessment process as part of an affiliated multidisciplinary group of external experts and consultants. This reviews project proposals; evaluates evidence; assists the dissemination of results and related HTA information; and proposes assessment topics. Currently, FinOHTA is undertaking a national project (Managed Uptake of Medical Methods – MUMM) to develop rules for the uptake of new medical technologies. FinOHTA is collaborating with 19 hospitals in Finland to gather input from clinicians and administrative decision-makers on the use of new medical technologies and potential topics for assessment (FinOHTA, 2006a). Additional visits and collaborative workshops are planned in order to devise recommendations and finalize a list of future assessment topics.

There is limited patient and public involvement in HTA activities affiliated with FinOHTA. The majority of investment in patient and public participation in assessments is made at the information dissemination stage (Lauslahti et al.,

2000). There has been discussion about collaborating with patient associations on the publication of patient guides and other educational materials.

Since 1995, over 70 research projects have been completed. The majority are systematic reviews (Eskola et al., 2004) undertaken by FinOHTA staff, external organizations and in collaboration with international assessment bodies (e.g. SBU). Examples of active and completed projects include:

- antimicrobial treatment strategies (1998-2006)
- glaucoma screening (2002-2004)
- colorectal cancer screening (2000)
- CE of treatment for otitis media in children (active)
- PSA screening for prostate cancer (active)
- orthodontics (2003-2006)
- telemedicine (2001, updated 2003).

FinOHTA has also supported several Cochrane Collaboration projects, including assessments of the effectiveness of psychoeducation and multi-professional rehabilitation in musculoskeletal diseases.

The PPB evaluates pharmaceuticals following applications in which manufacturers propose and justify their product's price (Jarvelin, 2002). Applications must include detailed and comprehensive information including the costs of the drug therapy, expected additional benefits (therapeutic and societal) and projected market penetration, all of which are supported on the basis of relevant clinical and health economic studies (Zentner et al., 2005). If a health economic evaluation is required,[39] manufacturers are required to submit an assessment of the costs and benefits of the product in comparison to alternative treatments, defined as either the most commonly used or best available treatment for a particular indication (Zentner et al., 2005). Ministry of Social Affairs and Health guidelines published in 1999 require manufacturers to use appropriate analysis methods (e.g. cost minimization, CE, cost-utility, cost-benefit) to outline all assumptions used in an evaluation; specify the target group for therapy and present any subgroup analyses; include direct and indirect costs (reported separately); use modelling to estimate health effects if necessary; and report incremental benefits and costs (ISPOR, 1999). In addition, all analyses should include a time horizon sufficient to permit evaluation of all the essential costs and health effects. All outcomes realized over one year or more

39. Health economic evaluation is required if the drug under review contains a new active substance or if otherwise required by the PPB.

are required to be discounted at both 0% and 5%, and sensitivity analyses should be included on variables of uncertainty (see Table A3.1).

As mandated by law, the PPB reviews applications for new drugs by considering the following factors in order to substantiate a "reasonable" wholesale price (Zentner et al., 2005):

- therapeutic benefit

- patient benefit

- health economic information (e.g. CE)

- comparison of wholesale prices of competitive products in Finland

- comparison of prices of the drug in other EU countries

- budget impact

- cost of manufacture – production and R&D.

A drug approved by the PPB qualifies automatically for inclusion in the basic reimbursement category, covering 50% of costs. Both the price and the reimbursement category are confirmed formally by the Secretariat of the PPB and Kela (Zentner et al., 2005). Applications for higher reimbursement levels (i.e. 75% and 100%) must demonstrate the product's usefulness and CE. A statement on the replacement or remedial effects of the product is also required for 100% reimbursement. Manufacturers must submit information on the therapeutic value of the drug; projected dosage; cost of treatment compared to existing products for the same condition; market forecast on the cost impact of higher reimbursement status; and an itemized statement on the costs and benefits of the treatment, especially in comparison to alternative medications and other therapies (Zentner et al., 2005). This information is reviewed by the PPB and affiliated expert groups, if necessary. New drugs are intended to remain in the basic reimbursement category for two years before they are considered for special reimbursement (Zentner et al., 2005).

The PPB's decisions are valid for a limited duration. Drugs with new agent properties or effects can be re-evaluated every three years; other pharmaceuticals are examined every five years (Zentner et al., 2005).

HTA dissemination and implementation

FinOHTA aims to change existing health-care practices through the dissemination and implementation of assessment results and other HTA-related information, where needed. In fact, information provision is the primary method by which FinOHTA influences the health-care system (FinOHTA, 2006a).

The target audience is quite broad, encompassing those who work in, or are affiliated to, health care; patients; consumers; and the Ministry of Social Affairs and Health. Moreover, the national media (e.g. TV, radio, newspapers) are conduits for information delivery and important audiences for the work conducted at and through FinOHTA (FinOHTA, 2006a).

The objective is to reach as wide an audience as possible so a variety of methods and media are employed to disseminate information. The principal means of dissemination are its own publications, including the bi-monthly newsletter *Impakti*, FinOHTA reports (results from internal research projects) and technology updates (translation of research results from other assessment bodies). *Impakti* contains summaries of HTA research projects and is distributed to all hospital districts, health-care providers and selected policy decision-makers (Lauslahti et al., 2000). The majority of reviews commissioned by FinOHTA are published in both English and Finnish.

Other information dissemination media include the web site; targeted communications on international HTA results to national experts; and publications in academic and medical journals (Lauslahti et al., 2000). Furthermore, FinOHTA participates in national and international conferences, such as meetings held by the Finnish Medical Association and various specialist societies, and organizes courses on evidenced-based medicine.

Findings from FinOHTA projects and manufacturer-sponsored economic evaluations (in the case of the PPB) are used to inform decision-making and priority-setting activities primarily related to reimbursement, pricing and clinical policy and practice via the promulgation of guidelines. The PPB's primary use of health economic information is for decisions on the pricing and reimbursement status of pharmaceutical products; the primary intent of FinOHTA's results is to change clinical or health-care practices, where necessary. However, while FinOHTA plays this pivotal role, it is not the primary body responsible for implementation of assessment results. Hospital districts, health-care centres, and medical and health organizations have the principal responsibility for employing HTA research in policy and planning decision-making (Lauslahti et a., 2000).

FinOHTA collaborates with Duodecim to develop clinical treatment (Current Care) guidelines for common diseases and health problems (Duodecim, 2006b): 25 guidelines were available in February 2006, another 29 are in the pipeline. By 2010, there are expected to be 100 published Current Care guidelines. The Current Care board selects most topics from suggestions by medical specialist societies. A group of experts (e.g. general practitioners, allied health professionals) systematically review all relevant literature on the selected topic, including FinOHTA assessments, based on criteria outlined by an internal Evidence-Based Medicine Working Group (Duodecim, 2006b). This evidence forms the basis of draft guidelines that are distributed to key stakeholders for review and revision. Final guidelines are made available to the public via the Internet, CD-ROMs, relevant medical journals and a portal for Finnish health-care professionals – *Terveysportti*.

The Centre for Pharmacotherapy Development (ROHTO), under the Ministry of Social Affairs and Health, employs health economic information to develop and promulgate guidelines (FinOHTA, 2006b). Specifically, ROHTO evaluates, summarizes and disseminates information on evidence-based, cost-effective pharmacotherapy. The main vehicles for dissemination are the Finnish Medical Journal (*Lääkärilehti*) and the ROHTO web site. Articles typically highlight evidence-based information about drugs and current trends or challenges in prescribing patterns.

There is significant support for guideline development in Finland, but the process can be improved. For example, few of the most recently published Current Care guidelines included an economic component although the health economic component typically involved a CE evaluation. Moreover, there is no existing research evidence on the effect of ROHTO's programme on prescribing practices or on how effectively the Current Care guidelines have been adopted in practice (FinOHTA, 2006b).

Both the PPB and FinOHTA have areas that require improvement. The PPB has faced increased demand for health economic evaluations to support reimbursement and pricing decisions, but authorities have allocated limited resources to health economics expertise in practice. Hence, the PPB board does not contain a health economist, nor has it invested in expertise in health economics. Moreover, the European Court of Justice ruled recently that the PPB's pricing and reimbursement system is too slow and lacks sufficient transparency, especially for decisions regarding the special reimbursement category (Pharma Industry Finland, 2004).

In 2004, FinOHTA conducted an evaluation of the centre's operations and published a report on future strategies and recommendations to improve the HTA process (Eskola et al., 2004). Consultation with stakeholder groups and staff identified weaknesses including a shortage of health economic professionals to conduct the assessments required; a need for increased opportunities for formal education in technology assessment and better integration and coordination between FinOHTA and other bodies (e.g. Current Care and ROHTO), especially with respect to pharmaceuticals; and greater focus on patients and consumers in the assessment process and as targets of HTA-related information.

Table A3.1. *Overview of HTA governance, processes and role in decision-making in Finland*

Finland

HTA governance & organization

Institutions/committees	PPB – reimbursement and pricing decisions. FinOHTA – primary national HTA body. Ministry of Social Affairs and Health – guides health and social services in Finland; defines related policy and legislation. STAKES – oversees FinOHTA, monitors health care and social services and related R&D activities.
Entities responsible for reviewing HTA evidence for priority-setting and decision-making	PPB. Hospital districts, health-care providers and the Ministry of Social Affairs and Health (in the case of FinOHTA).
HTA agenda-setting body(s)	Ministry of Social Affairs and Health/STAKES/ FinOHTA.
Areas for HTA	New pharmaceuticals (PPB); drugs, devices, procedures, organizational and support systems in health care (FinOHTA).
Reimbursement requirements and limitations	Wholesale price, determined by the PPB, must be deemed reasonable. Reimbursement levels are 50%, 75% or 100%, depending on the disease area and cost of the pharmaceutical. Restrictions can be imposed according to indication, severity of illness and patient population.
Stakeholder involvement	Medical and health-care professionals and experts, representatives from consumer associations, hospital managers, academics (FinOHTA). Limited patient and public involvement in the HTA process.
International collaboration	SBU and other Nordic HTA bodies, HTAi, INAHTA, EUR-ASSESS, Cochrane Collaboration, AGREE Collaboration, EUnetHTA and G-I-N.

(cont.)

Table A3.1. *(cont.)*

HTA topic selection & analytical design

Governance of topic selection	FinOHTA and STAKES.
Criteria for topic selection	FinOHTA: • public health impact • significance for national economy. PPB – dependent upon manufacturer submissions.
Criteria for assessment	Therapeutic benefit, patient benefit, CE, budget impact and R&D (PPB). Therapeutic benefit, CE, budget impact, public health impact, service requirements and social/legal/ethical considerations (FinOHTA).
Criteria outlined or publicly-available	Yes.
Analysis perspective	Societal.
Duration required to conduct assessments	1 year for complete HTA; few months for Rapid Reviews (FinOHTA).

Evidence requirements & assessment methods[40]

Documents required from manufacturer	All relevant clinical and health economic studies, with modelling, if necessary.
Systematic literature review and synthesis	Not available.
Unpublished data/ grey literature	Not available.
Preferred clinical study type/ evidence	Head-to-head RCTs.

---

40. Section applies primarily to the PPB.

Type of economic assessment preferred or required	Cost-minimization, CE, cost-utility, cost-benefit analyses.
Availability of guidelines outlining methodological requirements	Published by the Ministry of Social Affairs and Health.
Choice of comparator	Most frequently used therapy.
Specification of outcome variable	Not available.
Sub-group analyses	Yes.
Costs included in analysis	Direct and indirect.
Incremental analyses required	Yes.
Time horizon	Sufficient duration to perform appraisal of main costs and health effects.
Equity issues	Not stated.
Discounting	Both costs and benefits: 0% and 5%.
Modelling	If effectiveness data not available or not applicable. Modelling performed by manufacturers. All assumptions must be justified.
Sensitivity analyses	For primary assumptions or other uncertainties.
CE or willingness-to-pay threshold	No formal threshold.
Missing or incomplete data	Not available.
Support for methodological development	FinOHTA.

(cont.)

Table A3.1. *(cont.)*

HTA dissemination & implementation

Channels for HTA results dissemination	FinOHTA publications (Impakti, FinOHTA reports, technology updates, brochures); web site; targeted communication of HTA results to network of experts; education (courses, seminars); academic journals; other medical and public health associations.
Use of HTA results	Reimbursement and pricing (PPB). Guide clinical practice and health-care services (FinOHTA).
Evidence considered in decision-making	Therapeutic benefit, patient benefit, CE/cost-utility, budget impact, costs of product and associated R&D and manufacture (PPB).
Any reported obstacles to effective implementation	European Court of Justice ruled that the PPB's pricing and reimbursement system is too slow and not transparent enough. Recent FinOHTA study identified: shortage of HTA staff/professionals; insufficient training in HTA; lack of patient/consumer focus to assessments; and poor coordination between HTA agencies.
Formal processes to measure impact	Project proposals approved and commissioned by FinOHTA must have a plan for evaluation and follow-up (via surveys, registry research or other methodological approach).
Processes for re-evaluation or appeals	Re-evaluation every 3 years for pharmaceuticals with new agent/properties/effects; otherwise, every 5 years (PPB).
Accountability for stakeholder input	Primarily clinical experts – contribute input to selection of project proposals, evaluation of assessment results and topics for assessment (FInOHTA).
Transparent/public decision-making process	PPB could improve transparency, especially for decisions on the special reimbursement category.

Sources: FinOHTA, 2006a; Zentner et al., 2005; OECD, 2003; Jarvelin, 2002; Lauslahti et al., 2000; ISPOR, 1999.

Appendix 4. France

Overview of health-care and reimbursement systems

Health is a fundamental right under the French Constitution, therefore health protection and medical care is guaranteed to the entire population. The jurisdiction of the health-care system is divided between the state (parliament, government and various ministries), statutory health insurance funds and (to a lesser extent) local communities (Sandier et al., 2004).

Direction of the health-care system at state level is substantiated by the Act on Social Security Funding. Passed on an annual basis since 1996 (Sandier et al., 2004), this is based on reports of the Social Security Accounts Commission and the National Health Conference.[41] It sets projected targets for health-insurance spending, reports on health policy and social security trends and delineates any new provisions concerning benefits and regulation (Sandier et al., 2004).

A significant level of control lies with the Ministry of Health and its directorates of general health and policy, hospital and health care, social security and of social policy. The Ministry also controls a significant portion of the regulation of health-care expenditure on the basis of the overall framework established by Parliament. Key areas of responsibility include allocating budgeted expenditure to different health-care sectors; approving agreements between health insurance funds and relevant unions; establishing prices of specific medical procedures and drugs; and defining priority areas for national health programmes (Sandier et al., 2004).

Over the last ten years, the state has established a number of independent committees and agencies to fulfil specific functions and lend specialized expertise, including the following key authorities (Bellanger et al., 2005; Sandier et al., 2004; Fleurette & Banta, 2000).

- *High Committee for Public Health.* Established in 1991 within the Ministry of Health. Provides guidance and assists decision-making on public-health problems and issues related to the organization of health-care delivery.

- *Agency for Medical Safety of Food Products (AFSSA).* Under the Ministry of Health, evaluates nutritional and health risks in foods and conducts research in these areas.

---

41. Annual National Health Conference proposes priorities and suggests policy directions to government and parliament. Comprises mainly health-care professionals and representatives from health-care organizations and regional health councils.

- *National Institute for Monitoring Public Health (InVS).* Monitors the population's public heath, especially in the areas of communicable diseases, environmental health, health at work, and chronic diseases.

- *French Agency for Medical Safety of Health Products (AFSSAPS).* Under the Ministry of Health, responsible for overseeing the safety of health products.

- *National Agency for Accreditation and Evaluation of Health (ANAES).* Instituted in 1997 to create and disseminate practice guidelines, promote clinicians' education and professional development, accredit hospitals and provide guidance on procedures eligible for reimbursement from the health insurance funds. Comprises physicians, other health-care professionals and economists. Overall agenda set by Board of Directors, Ministry of Health, health insurance funds and medical unions. High Health Authority replaced ANAES under the Health Insurance Act 2004 (see Box A4.1).

- *Economic Committee on Health Products (CEPS).* Inter-ministerial committee that sets prices for drugs and medical devices and monitors trends in pharmaceutical spending in relation to annual budget targets.

The Ministry of Social Affairs, Labour and Solidarity and the social security, health, and hospitals and health care directorates also have some jurisdiction over the French health-care system. In general, these bodies operate a powerful top-down approach to decision- and policy-making.

Box A4.1. High Health Authority in France

The High Health Authority (*Haute Authorité de Santé*) was created by the Health Insurance Act 2004. The Authority serves as an independent scientific public authority with legal status. Its principal objective is to evaluate the medical usefulness of medical procedures, services and products that are reimbursed by the health insurance funds. The Authority has four main functions.

- Devise recommendations on reimbursement conditions for health-care procedures, especially for certain diseases.

- Provide medical and public health expertise to support reimbursement-related decision-making.

- Distribute guidelines to health-care professionals and the general public.

- Develop and implement hospital accreditation procedures and requirements.

The High Health Authority works closely with the French Health Products Safety Agency (Afssaps) and the Institute for Public Health Surveillance (InVS).

Statutory health insurance (SHI) is the second level of health-care jurisdiction. A branch of the wider social security system, this system provides almost universal insurance coverage to the French population. It comprises three principal schemes determined by an individual's social and/or professional category (Bellanger et al., 2005; Sandier et al., 2004). The general scheme (*régime général*) covers employees and pensioners from trade and industry, and their families (approximately 84% of the population). It is financed mainly by payroll contributions from both employers and employees. The agricultural scheme covers farmers and agricultural workers (and their families); the scheme for non-agricultural self-employed people covers craftsmen and self-employed individuals. Together these two cover approximately 12% of the population. Other schemes cover certain categories of the population on an employment-related basis. Several are associated with the general scheme (e.g. those for civil servants, physicians working under health insurance agreements, students and military personnel) (Sandier et al., 2004).

The SHI funds about 75% of total health spending. A significant proportion of the French population is affiliated with voluntary, supplementary sickness funds or purchases private insurance to complement SHI (Bellanger et al., 2005); approximately 85% of the population is covered under complementary health insurance.

The Social Security Directorate directs the health insurance system under the Ministry of Health. However, various regional institutions collaborate with the Ministry to oversee health services and the three main insurance schemes. These bodies serve both strategic and operational roles in health-service delivery and financing throughout the country (Bellanger et al., 2005).

The French insurance system offers expansive reimbursement within the areas of preventive, curative, rehabilitative and palliative care. In particular, reimbursable medical products and services include hospital care, outpatient treatment, diagnostic services, pharmaceutical products and medical devices and prescribed health-care-related transport. However, the reimbursement of such goods and services depends on their registration in positive lists (Bellanger et al., 2005). In order to be eligible for SHI reimbursement pharmaceuticals must be on the *Liste de Spécialités Pharmaceutiques Remboursables aux Assurés Sociaux* (LSPRAS); medical devices and related services on the *Liste des Produits et Prestations Remboursables* (LPP); and medical procedures on the *Classification Commune des Actes Medicaux* (CCAM) (Bellanger et al., 2005). Moreover, all medical products and services must be prescribed by health-care professionals (e.g. physicians, midwives, dentists) and in the appropriate medical context (Bellanger et al., 2005).

Before the Health Insurance Act, positive lists were enforced by the relevant ministries, including the inclusion of new goods and services (Bellanger et al., 2005). Ministers based their decisions on the advice of various ad-hoc commissions and agencies, especially ANAES. Since August 2004 the National Union of Health Insurance Funds (*Union Nationale des Caisses d'Assurance Maladie* – UNCAM), represented by all three health insurance funds, has defined the positive lists for pharmaceuticals, procedures and medical devices[42] (Bellanger et al., 2005). The High Health Authority assumed responsibility for the Transparency Commission (Commission de la Transparence, described in further detail below) when it replaced ANAES. The Authority assists UNCAM's decision-making by providing advice and recommendations on the positive list, as does the Union of Voluntary Health Insurers (*Union Nationale des Organismes d'Assurance Maladie Complémentaire* – UNOC), also created by the 2004 Act.

All pharmaceutical products must undergo a three stage process prior to registration for reimbursement (Sandier et al., 2004).

1. Afssaps evaluates a drug for effectiveness, safety and quality before granting market authorization.

2. Authorized products are reviewed for inclusion on the positive list of reimbursable drugs. The manufacturer must submit a request for inclusion (accompanied by a suggested price).[43] Approval for inclusion and determination of the reimbursement rate is established by a health and social security ministerial order based on review and recommendation by the Transparency Commission of the High Health Authority (see HTA procedures and processes below).

3. Transparency Commission advice on the relative therapeutic value and costs of a drug is sent to CEPS, which negotiates the price with the manufacturer. The price is based on a number of factors including therapeutic benefit (compared to other listed products in the same therapeutic class), price of similar drugs, projected sales volume and estimated utilization. Following substantiation of an agreed price, a drug can be included in the positive list.

The Transparency Commission consists of 31 members (including a president) representing the government, statutory health insurance system and medical and pharmaceutical experts (Zentner et al., 2005). As of 2005, approximately

---

42. UNCAM is also responsible for setting rates for medical procedures, drugs and devices, and for determining co-payment and co-insurance levels.

43. A drug does not have to be reimbursable in order to be prescribed in France. Manufacturers can decide not to seek reimbursement in order to retain freedom of pricing.

1340 recommendations on new pharmaceuticals had been officially published by the Commission.

No one organization is responsible for systematic evaluation of medical devices, but manufacturers must apply for official reimbursement before they can be used in private institutions[44] (Orvain et al., 2004). The reimbursement review process conducted by the Product and Services Evaluation Commission (CEPP) entails an evaluation of the product (Bellanger et al., 2005). The procedures (i.e. assessment and criteria) are similar to those applied to drugs. Chaired by Afssaps, CEPP comprises scientific experts as well as representatives of the health insurance funds and device manufacturers, overseen by the Ministries of Health and of Social Security.

HTA governance and organization

In the 1970s, growing concern about the quality and efficiency of health care led to increased awareness of the need for HTA to evaluate medical practice or health technology and develop priorities. The Government established the National Committee for Medical Evaluation in Health Care in 1987 [45] and, two years later, a non-profit, independent association – the National Agency for the Development and Evaluation of Medicines (ANDEM) (Fleurette & Banta, 2000). ANDEM was to lead all health-care and technology assessment programmes (except pharmaceuticals) with the objective of providing the Ministry of Health and the health insurance funds with scientific evidence on the safety, effectiveness and CE of health technologies. This remit involved developing internal HTA projects; validating the methods and funding of external research; and disseminating results and other relevant information (Fleurette & Banta, 2000). Assessment topics were identified by the Ministry of Health, health insurance funds, ANDEM's board of directors and scientific council and other relevant professional groups. The association's staff was comprised mostly of physicians, these consulted with many external scientific experts and health professionals. The Board of Directors included representatives of the Ministries of Health, Education, Research and of Agriculture and Fisheries.

At ANDEM, assessments typically involved a method of combined critical appraisal of published literature with expert and professional consultation (Orvain et al., 2004). ANDEM published over 30 reports including evaluation of bone-density measurement (1991); assessment of cochlear implants (1994); silicone breast implants (1996); and implantable cardioverter defibrillators

---

44. Not necessary for use in public hospitals.

45. The Committee lacked a budget and any official agenda but discussed mainly ethical issues and methods of evaluation in health care.

(1997). ANDEM was also involved in consensus conferences, clinical practice guidelines and evaluation activities in the public and private hospital sectors (e.g. clinical audits and quality assurance programmes).

In 1996, ANDEM was replaced by the ANAES and most technology assessments of medical devices were moved from ANDEM to Afssaps. The inclusion of all medical procedures on the positive list depended on the advice of ANAES until 2004 when it was replaced by the High Health Authority (Ballenger et al., 2005). In addition, ANAES was actively involved in consensus conferences to develop standards for practice appraisal and guidance development (Orvain et al., 2004).

Several other organizations in France are involved in HTA activities (Ballenger et al., 2005; Sandier et al., 2004; Fleurette & Banta, 2000).

- *French National Institute for Health and Medical Research* (Inserm). Specializes in biomedical and public health research, including evaluation projects.

- *Committee for Evaluation and Diffusion of Innovative Technologies* (CEDIT). Established in 1982 as an advisory body for the Hospitals of Paris General Director, primarily to assist in decision-making regarding investments in new and costly medical technologies. Similar committees are, or have been, developed at other hospitals.

- *French Health Economists Association* (CES). In collaboration with Inserm developed an analytical database (CODECS) on health economic evaluations and related research.

- *Various academic institutions.* Public health departments and medical schools are developing courses and research activity in economic evaluation.

- *Private consultancy firms.* A number of consulting companies have established practice areas related to health-care evaluation and hospital management.

HTA processes and procedures[46]

It is presumed that the High Health Authority has assumed many of the processes and procedures employed by its predecessor. ANAES prioritized topics for HTA reports following a customer consultation process and defined priorities and the annual HTA programme via a postal survey of assessment needs (Orvain et al., 2004). Responses were evaluated according to:

- extent of public health issue

---

46. Evaluation processes for reimbursement and pricing decisions focus on the Transparency Commission/CEP and CEPP.

- variability in practice

- disease prevalence

- characteristics of the patient population

- availability of supporting data

- novelty or innovation of the technology

- underlying policy or clinical question.

After this review, experts on particular topics might be interviewed and consulted and the type of report required was determined – full report, rapid assessment or brief update. A work-plan was prepared and presented to ANAES's scientific council, which selected topics by various voting methods. The Administrative Board subsequently approved the complete programme. Since 1999, important topics have included imaging technologies; emerging therapeutic and diagnostic techniques; and public heath issues (Orvain et al., 2004).

An ANAES HTA programme typically comprised two principal types of assessment: (i) evidence-based assessments of widely used technology and of new technology prior to dissemination and (ii) rapid assessments of innovative or fast-developing technologies, or emerging public health issues. ANAES typically followed a standardized procedure for HTA assessment, as outlined in Box A4.2.

Box A4.2. Procedures for a standard HTA at ANAES

- Systematic literature search.

- Articles selected by pre-established criteria.

- Expert working group established to validate study design and provide expertise.

- Health economist (or team) systematically appraises literature and prepares draft report addressing technical aspects, effectiveness and CE, where possible.

- Working group reviews draft report and provides recommendations and revisions.

- Reviewers (from various stakeholder groups and backgrounds) comment on amended report.

- Report approved following any necessary revisions and vetting by the Scientific Council.

- Full report published and posted on ANAES web site; summaries disseminated; press conferences convened; and articles published.

Source: Orvain et al., 2004.

Most ANAES assessments were based on systematic review of evidence, but a range of methods was introduced, such as expert panels and modelling.

The Transparency Commission and CEPS' assessments for the reimbursement of pharmaceuticals in France are contingent on two primary factors. Products must contribute to either an improvement in the prescribed treatment, relative to other drugs in the same therapeutic class, or a decrease in the cost of treatment (Sandier et al., 2004). Since 1999 the Transparency Commission has been required to confirm these outcomes by conducting an evaluation of therapeutic benefit (*Amelioration du Service Medical Rendu* – ASMR)(Sandier et al., 2004). Manufacturers submit clinical studies and related data to the Commission for review; a comparative health economic analysis is not required (for further detail see Table A4.1).

Pharmacoeconomic evidence is used principally to determine the financial impact of a drug and inform pricing decisions (Zentner et al., 2005)). A group of experts in economic evaluation, appointed by the directors of CEPS and Afssaps, advises on the quality of evidence and methods used in the pharmacoeconomic studies (Bellanger et al., 2005; Zentner et al., 2005). These experts are required to have no links with the pharmaceutical industry or the particular product sponsor. CEPS and Afssaps provide guidelines to manufacturers on pharmacoeconomic study requirements (Zentner et al., 2005). Additional information is collected regarding the therapeutic situations in which a product should be used most appropriately and the projected size of the patient population.

The Commission reviews available evidence and evaluates a product across a variety of criteria, including (Zentner et al., 2005):

• effectiveness of a drug and possible side effects;

• therapeutic value relative to other available treatments (yes/no classification for existence of therapeutic alternatives);

• severity of disease or condition;

• clinical profile of the drug (curative, preventive, symptomatic properties);

• public health impact.

Having applied these criteria, the therapeutic value (the SMR) is evaluated for each indication across six levels (Zentner et al., 2005; Bellanger et al., 2005).

1. Significant therapeutic benefit.

2. Considerable therapeutic benefit, in terms of efficacy and side effect profile.

3. Moderate therapeutic benefit, in terms of efficacy and side-effect profile; existing product, where equivalent pharmaceuticals exist.

4. Minor improvement in terms of efficacy and/or utility.

5. No improvement, but still recommended for positive list due to lower associated costs.

6. Unsuitable for inclusion on the reimbursement list.

In addition to new therapies, between 1999 and 2001 all existing pharmaceuticals on the positive list were reclassified according to the SMR criteria.

UNCAM reviews the ASMR and decides whether the drug can be included on the positive list. Typically, the costs of a drug are not considered when reimbursement status is determined. However, costs of a new therapy are considered for me-too products and generic alternatives. These may be reimbursed if the new therapy's costs are lower than existing alternatives (Anell, 2004). Also, the Commission's assessment must define any restrictive conditions (e.g. prescription limitations) regarding the reimbursement of new and expensive pharmaceuticals.[47]

The SMR level and the severity of disease determine the reimbursement rate for each product (Sandier et al., 2004). Pharmaceuticals are granted 35%, 65% or 100% coverage (Zentner et al., 2005). The lower rate of reimbursement generally applies to drugs used for more typical, less serious conditions; the higher rate applies to products used to treat life-threatening or chronic conditions (e.g. diabetes, AIDS, cancer). Approximately half of the drugs available on the market in France are included on the positive list of reimbursable drugs; the majority within the 35% rate (Bellanger et al., 2005).

While UNCAM makes the final judgment on the inclusion or exclusion of goods and services from the positive list, the Ministers of Health and Social Security have the right to reject these decisions, especially where public health issues are concerned (Bellanger et al. 2005). The Ministers are allowed one month to decline UNCAM's recommendations and provide their justification for doing so. Before the 2004 Act, ministers had several months in which to make decisions with no requirement for explanations.

Decisions about the price of reimbursable pharmaceuticals are determined by negotiations between CEPS and the manufacturers.[48] These negotiations

---

47. Usually outlined in a specific document – the FIT (*Fiche d'Information Therapeutic*).

48. Typically held privately. Reasons for conclusions are not disclosed.

are based on the Transparency Commission's ASMR, particularly the SMR classification, and the following factors (Bellanger et al., 2005; Sandier et al., 2004):

- relevance of the respective product in the pharmaceutical market (evaluated by expected sales volume);

- research expenditure;

- manufacturer's advertising costs.

A manufacturer who claims a price premium for a new, innovative product is required to supply supporting evidence, such as clear clinical improvement over similar existing products. Moreover, pharmaceuticals that are therapeutic breakthroughs, and therefore without competition, are compared internationally in order to negotiate the price between state and manufacturer (Zentner et al., 2005). However, there is no formal mechanism for setting the price of a drug in France on the basis of its price in other European countries. Prices of reimbursable drugs may not be changed without the authorization of CEPS (Bellanger et al., 2005).

Inclusion on the positive list lasts for five years and essentially fixes the statutory reimbursement price (Zentner et al., 2005). However, if there are changes in the therapeutic standards the Transparency Commission can reassess the SMR at any time. Normally, the five-year re-evaluation takes account of all current studies and the product's application in clinical practice (Zentner et al., 2005). Prescription profiles are analysed in order to assess whether the drug has been prescribed correctly before it can be restored to the positive list.

The assessment procedures and criteria for reimbursement of medical devices are similar to those applied to drugs (Bellanger et al., 2005; Sandier et al., 2004). The preliminary review procedures for medical devices are undertaken by CEPP. These include a description of the product or service; assessment of the SMR; therapeutic and diagnostic criteria for inclusion on the positive list (if necessary); and the types of prescription and use of the medical device required for reimbursement (Bellanger et al., 2005). CEPP is also responsible for any additional SMR assessments related to a product's renewal on the positive list. Reimbursement rates for medical devices vary from 65% to 100%, depending on the SMR rating (Bellanger et al., 2005). As for drugs, CEPS bases the reference pricing on its own report and information from manufacturers.

HTA dissemination and implementation

All reimbursable pharmaceuticals and medical devices on the positive list are published and publicly available in the official journals of the Ministers of Health and Social Security and CEPS.

Bellanger et al. (2005) report that the determination of the positive list is a contentious issue in France, especially among those in the Ministries of Health and Social Security. French health policy promotes regulation harmonization and health equality. However, these objectives must be implemented in, but are ultimately hampered by, a context of increasing health expenditures and user fees. Moreover, while regulation of the positive list and benefits package is explicit, the coverage of particular aspects of patient care remains somewhat implicit. (Bellanger et al., 2005). It may be that not all goods and services are covered to the same extent in practice.

It remains to be seen whether the delegation of decision-making responsibilities for the benefits package to two self-governing bodies (High Health Authority and UNCAM) is fully effective. Historically, both the French Government and physicians have held significant power in the health-care decision-making process. The Ministers of Health and Social Security still retain rights to reject any of UNCAM's decisions.

ANAES uses assessment results primarily to advise on prospective clinical or economic research and on resource requirements (e.g. equipment or staff needs). ANAES has a minimal formal role in decision- and policy-making so those who commission the reports have no statutory obligation to accept or consider its recommendations. Orvain et al. (2004) pointed out several factors other than economic evaluation that influence decisions e.g. budget, social factors and political priorities. Consequently, the impact of HTA assessments depends heavily on the implementation by the end decision-maker or the user of the recommendations.

However, many ANAES reports have made an impact on many different levels of decision-making and clinical practice. Two years after an ANAES recommendation against mass prostate-cancer screening, the Ministry of Health requested confirmation. ANAES's re-evaluation of available evidence and reaffirmation of the original conclusions was upheld by the Ministry. While this example supports the use of HTA in decision-making, it remains uncertain how these reports were taken into account during the process.

Table A4.1. *Overview of HTA governance, processes and role in decision-making in France*

France

HTA governance & organization

Institutions/committees	Transparency Commission.
	CEPS.
	CEPP.
	All three work under the auspices of the High Health Authority.
Entities responsible for reviewing HTA evidence for priority-setting and decision-making	Transparency Commission/CEPS and CEPP/ CEPS.
	UNCAM.
	Ministry of Health and Ministry of Social Security.
HTA agenda-setting body(s)	Products for assessment selected by manufacturers' applications for registration on the positive list.
Areas for HTA	Pharmaceuticals and medical devices.
Reimbursement requirements and limitations	Therapeutic benefit and improved side-effect profile relative to similar products on the positive list; decrease in cost of treatment.
Stakeholder involvement	Medical, scientific and pharmaceutical experts; physicians and other health professionals.
International collaboration	EUnetHTA, G-I-N, INAHTA, International Society for Quality in Health Care.

HTA topic selection & analytical design

Governance of topic selection	For Transparency Commission/CEP and CEPP, dependent upon manufacturer's submission.
Criteria for topic selection	For Transparency Commission/CEP and CEPP, dependent upon manufacturer's submission.

Criteria for assessment	Products evaluated across the following criteria:

- effectiveness of drug and possible side effects
- position in the therapeutic spectrum relative to other available treatments
- disease or condition severity
- clinical profile of the drug
- public health impact.

Criteria outlined or publicly-available	Yes.
Analysis perspective	Depends on the purpose of the assessment/ study.

Evidence requirements & assessment methods[49]

Documents required from manufacturer	Clinical studies.
Systematic literature review and synthesis	Yes.
Unpublished data/ grey literature	Not available.
Preferred clinical study type/ evidence	Double-blind head-to-head RCTs.
Type of economic assessment preferred or required	Any one of cost-minimization, CE, cost-utility or cost-benefit analysis. Choice must be justified.
Availability of guidelines outlining methodological requirements	CEPS and Afssaps provide guidelines to manufacturers on pharmacoeconomic study requirements.
Choice of comparator	Approved, listed pharmaceuticals of the same therapeutic category, in terms of those:

- used most regularly (by treatment days)
- with the cheapest treatment costs
- included in the positive list most recently.

(cont.)

---

49. Section applies primarily to the Transparency Commission, CEPP and CEPS.

Table A4.1. *(cont.)*

Specification of outcome variable	Final outcomes preferred: mortality, morbidity and quality of life.
Sub-group analyses	Amongst other patient groups; extent and severity of illness; and co-morbidities. A priori definition must be established.
Costs included in analysis	Depends on the aim of the study/assessment. All relevant costs must be reported and presented in detail. Indirect costs must be reported separately.
Incremental analyses required	Yes.
Time horizon	Long enough to capture long-term effects and costs.
Equity issues	Not stated.
Discounting	Costs and benefits 2.5%-5%. Outcomes must be presented with and without discounting.
Modelling	Sufficient detail and justification required.
Sensitivity analyses	On main variables of uncertainty. Sufficient detail and reporting required.
CE or willingness-to-pay threshold	No formal threshold.
Missing or incomplete data	Not available.
Support for methodological development	No.

HTA dissemination & implementation

Duration required to conduct assessments	Few months.
Channels for HTA results dissemination	Official journals of Ministers of Health and Social Security and CEPS.
Use of HTA results	Reimbursement and pricing decisions.
Evidence considered in decision-making	Clinical, epidemiological and economic data; financial and public health impact.
Any reported obstacles to effective implementation	Not available.
Formal processes to measure impact	Not available.
Processes for re-evaluation or appeals	Mandatory re-evaluation process every five years.
Accountability for stakeholder input	ANAES: various stakeholders identify priorities for assessment and comment on draft reports. Patient participation is limited, if not non-existent.
Transparent/public decision-making process	Input required from various decision-making bodies: Transparency Commission, CEPS, CEPP, UNCAM and Ministries of Health and Social Services. Ministers have discretion to reject recommendations regarding the positive list, all decisions must be made within one month and justified explicitly. Pricing negotiations and conclusions are not made public.

Sources: Bellanger et al., 2005; Zentner et al., 2005; Sandier et al., 2004; OECD, 2003; Fleurette & Banta, 2000.

Appendix 5. Germany

Overview of health-care and reimbursement systems

Shared decision-making processes between the *Lander*,[50] the Government and civil society organizations are a central tenet of German political structure, especially for the health-care system (Busse et al., 2005). While the Federal Government, Federal Assembly and the Federal Council have assumed increasing responsibility for health-care reform and legislation since the 1980s, still the health-care system is characterized by a relatively high level of decentralization and independent decision-making. In particular, the Government typically delegates responsibilities to membership-based, independent payer and provider organizations involved with the financing and delivery of health care covered by the social insurance schemes, notably the SHI. Such entities are self-regulated, with mandatory membership and internal control of decisions on membership fees and the delivery and financing of health services (Busse et al., 2005). Joint committees of payers and providers have the mandate to define benefits, rights and prices (at federal level); negotiate contracts; and control and sanction members (at regional level).

Other entities (such as health-provider associations, patient organizations and private health insurance bodies) contribute to the decision-making and priority-setting process via consultation, shared financing of health-care provision, advocacy and the submission of proposals (Busse et al., 2005). The German Constitution defines areas of exclusive federal and concurrent legislation (Busse et al., 2005). Health does not fall under an area of excusive federal legislation, but specific health issues are included in concurrent legislation, such as infectious diseases that threaten public safety, pharmaceuticals and the economy of hospitals. The *Lander* is responsible for all primary aspects of public health but is superseded by federal law, where it exists.

The Federal Assembly, Federal Council and the Ministry for Health (BMG)[51] are key actors at federal level. The BMG is responsible for eight principal areas including: European and international social and health policy; pharmaceuticals and health protection; health care, SHI, and long-term care; and disease prevention, control and biomedicine. It collaborates with several subordinate authorities for licensing and supervisory functions and for consultation on scientific and technical matters.

---

50. The 16 states that comprise the Federal Republic of Germany.

51. Ministry of Health and Social Security prior to 2005.

- *Federal Institute for Drugs and Medical Devices (BfArM).* Licenses pharmaceuticals and ensures the safety of pharmaceuticals and medical devices.

- *German Institute of Medical Documentation and Information (DIMDI).* Responsible for providing public and relevant professionals with scientific and technical information on health care and medicine. Since 2000, has organized, coordinated and published HTA reports. Also maintains several large health-care related databases.

- *Federal Institute for Infectious and Non-Infectious Diseases.* Oversees surveillance, detection, prevention and control of diseases. Responsible for disseminating reports and epidemiological bulletins to the public and professionals. Also coordinates all activities related to infectious-disease control.

- *Federal Centre for Health Education (BZgA).* Develops and distributes health education materials and information. Also organizes, coordinates and supports prevention campaigns and social-marketing research.

Other relevant bodies at federal level include the Federal Social Insurance Authority and the Federal Financial Supervisory Authority (BaFin), responsible for national social insurance and private, for-profit insurance, respectively.

The majority of the 16 state governments at *Lander* level are involved in health matters, usually in collaboration with the Ministry of Labour and Social Affairs. This body houses several different divisions responsible for the following health-related areas (Busse et al., 2005):

- public health services[52]

- health promotion and prevention, AIDS treatment

- state-owned hospitals

- hospital planning

- supervision of health professionals and associated institutions

- pharmaceuticals and supervision of pharmacists.

The provider side of the SHI scheme is overseen by affiliated physician and other health-professional associations. The Federal Association of SHI Physicians is responsible for coordinating the organizational and federal levels.

---

52. Although public health services differ across *Lander*, they typically include health reporting, surveillance of communicable diseases, supervision of hospitals, health education and promotion, and oversight of commercial activities, including pharmaceuticals and foods.

Moreover, there is at least one provider association within each of the *Lander*. The purchaser side comprises independent sickness funds and related entities organized on a regional and/or federal basis. As of January 2004, there were 292 statutory funds, accounting for approximately 72 million insured people (Busse et al., 2005). The sickness funds have a statutory remit to decide the contribution levels of their members.

Germany follows a pluralistic funding scheme. The major source of health-care financing is SHI (by way of sickness funds), covering more than 85% of the population; private health insurance;[53] and other, sector-oriented governmental (e.g. military) schemes. All members and their dependents are entitled to comparable benefits regardless of insurance status, contribution levels or duration of coverage. These benefits are outlined in the Social Code Book (Busse & Riesberg, 2004). The breadth of benefits offered typically includes prevention and health promotion activities; treatment of diseases (e.g. ambulatory medical care, pharmaceuticals, medical devices and home nursing care); screening; emergency care; and patient education. While the Social Code Book regulates preventive services and screening, the Federal Joint Committee has considerable discretion in defining the benefits package, especially for pharmaceuticals and diagnostic and therapeutic procedures.

Unlike many European countries Germany does not have a positive list for drugs or other medical technologies, although several attempts were made to introduce this throughout the 1990s and early 2000s. Until 2003, market registration equated to blanket SHI coverage (and private health insurance reimbursement) with a few exceptions such as drugs for minor conditions (e.g. common cold); products deemed "inefficient" and therefore contained on a negative list; and therapies limited to certain indications (Busse & Reisberg, 2004). However, additional exclusions have been introduced by the implementation of the Statutory Health Insurance Modernization Act 2004, including lifestyle (Federal Joint Committee has full discretion to define this restriction) and OTC drugs for use by persons over 12 years old (Busse & Reisberg, 2004). The Act also introduced new stipulations for off-label drug use.

The decision-making powers of SHI bodies have decreased in most European countries as a result of cost-containment concerns, but Germany counters this trend. The Federal Government's aim to exercise more control over the benefits

---

53. Private health insurance predominantly offers either full coverage to a portion of the population or supplements SHI. Individuals with full coverage are typically active or retired public employees (e.g. teachers), self-employed individuals, or employed persons that opt out of SHI due to income considerations. Approximately 10% of the German population is covered by private insurance.

package has translated into increased state responsibility for decisions by the independent SHI entities, primarily via joint committees (Busse & Reisberg, 2004). Federal legislation has promoted competition on the provision of services while centralizing decision-making powers for the benefits basket.

Since the 2004 Act, various joint committees on ambulatory care, the hospital sector and services coordination have been combined in the Federal Joint Committee (Busse et al., 2005). Based on legislative mandate, this committee issues directives on all sectors of care, including HTA and pharmaceuticals. For pharmaceuticals, the directives encompass a broad range of decisions on coverage, clinical guidelines and price determination for outpatient drugs covered by the SHI. The Committee provides information on the efficacy, safety and prices of products by indication and promulgates practice guidelines according to relative benefits and price rather than excluding drugs from SHI coverage (Busse & Reisberg, 2004; Busse et al., 2005). It is also responsible for determining products subject to the reference pricing scheme.[54]

All directives issued by the Federal Joint Committee are transferred to the BMG for final recommendation. However, most of its decision-making processes are complemented by the Institute for Quality and Efficiency (IQWiG), an independent foundation to support evidence-based decision-making in Germany. This produces evidence-based reports on topics requested by the Federal Joint Committee and the BMG, and coordinates and publishes scientific work in various areas (see *HTA process and procedures* below). It has responsibility for:

- evaluating the safety and efficacy of drugs to determine inclusion in the reference pricing scheme;

- developing reports on the quality and efficiency of the health-benefits package;

- providing recommendations on disease-management programmes;

- assessing evidence-based guidelines for epidemiological conditions;

- disseminating reports to the public regarding the quality and efficiency of health care;

- evaluating and reporting on current knowledge regarding new and innovative diagnostic and therapeutic interventions for select diseases.

The IQWiG internal steering committee includes the director and several departmental leaders and has the aim of developing and maintaining the

---

54. Since 2004, for both patented and off-patent drugs.

methods of the institute. IQWiG is funded through the national health insurance scheme and is overseen by the BMG.

Review and accountability of decisions made by not only the Federal Joint Committee but also other single and joint committees on the corporate/ organizational level, is undertaken by the independent committees and entities themselves, the Federal Government (via the BMG) and the social courts (Busse & Riesberg, 2004). Self-regulation has been supported as it provides a foundation for effective negotiations, public trust and safeguards against excessive and unwarranted government involvement. It has also been criticized for lacking transparency and accountability.

HTA governance and organization

Historically, neither the control of health technology nor the use of HTA have been prominent issues for Germany, despite the need for evidence-based decision-making (Perleth & Busse, 2000). German regulations, especially those for licensing pharmaceuticals and medical devices, meet international standards but other types of therapies and certain aspects of health technology use and diffusion have not received sufficient attention. Increased awareness among decision-makers (primarily the Government and self-governing bodies) about the need for HTA to support decision-making on different levels of health care and to enhance networking on a European level and various health-care reforms, has served to strengthen and institutionalize HTA in Germany.

Prior to the early 2000s, coverage decisions and the management of health technology use and diffusion in Germany showed considerable inconsistence between different health-care sectors. For instance, the ambulatory sector was notably more regulated than the hospital sector, where explicit coverage decisions were virtually non-existent[55] (Busse & Reisberg, 2004). The difference(s) between sectors constituted a barrier to regulation and to HTA's role as an effective mechanism for informed decision-making and priority-setting. The SHI Reform Act 2000 was aimed at addressing this and strengthening HTA within the health-care system by establishing a new unit within DIMDI – the German Agency for Health Technology Assessment (DAHTA). This develops HTA reports and covers a range of other activities, including maintaining a database-support information system on health-care interventions. The information system offers access to national and international databases and to scientific evidence in the HTA field.

---

55. Primarily because coverage of medical devices and expensive medical equipment falls under budget negotiations at hospital level and hospital plans at state level.

Two leadership boards support DAHTA. The HTA Board of Trustees comprises representatives of self-governing bodies in the German health system, consumer groups and industry. Its principal task is to determine and select topics for HTA reports. The Scientific Advisory Board comprises medical and health economic experts, and primarily contributes to methodological issues during the assessment process.

As described, IQWiG supports the Federal Joint Committee's decisions on therapies and measures to be financed by SHI, among other activities related to HTA.

The entities listed below are also involved in HTA activities (Busse et al., 2005; Busse & Reisberg, 2004; Perleth & Busse, 2000).

- *Office of Technology Assessment at the German Parliament (TAB).* Established in 1990 as an independent scientific institution to support the German Parliament's decision-making on research and technology. Primary activities include designing and implementing HTA projects and monitoring major scientific and related social trends. Currently moving towards expanding its range of activities by contributing to long-term technology projects and analysing international policies and innovation developments.

- *Institute for Technology Assessment and Systems Analysis (ITAS).* Involved in a wide range of endeavours including technology assessment, socioeconomic environmental research and risk assessment. Supported by the Ministry of Education and Research; Ministry for the Environment, Nature Conservation and Nuclear Safety; and the EU Commission.

- *Institute for Medical Outcome Research (IMOR).* Contributes to the planning and conduct of clinical trials, meta-analyses, health economic studies and medical decision-making.

- *Potsdam Institute of Pharmacoepidemiology and Technology Assessment.* Examines the epidemiology of drug effects and utilization and provides education on pharmacoepidemiology and HTA.

- *German Scientific Working Group of Technology Assessment in Health Care.* Established as result of BMG initiative to stimulate HTA activities in Germany for improved decision-making at federal and corporate levels. Remit includes maintaining an HTA database (in collaboration with DAHTA), piloting evaluations of select medical technologies and standardizing methods for technology assessment. In addition, exchanges information about priorities for future assessments of health technologies with the Federal Joint Committee.

HTA process and procedures

The HTA process at DAHTA is fairly standardized and guided by institutionalized standard operating procedures (SOPs) that outline the steps to be followed during the scope of an assessment. These were developed and based on internal expertise and the experiences of other international HTA agencies, such as the Agency for Healthcare Research and Quality (AHRQ) in the United States, the Canadian Agency for Drugs and Technologies in Health (CADTH) and NCCHTA in the United Kingdom.

Topics for HTA reports can be nominated by a variety of stakeholders (including the BMG) and entered into a database via a questionnaire available on the DAHTA web site. Proposals can suggest clinical topics as well as methodical questions of HTA, evidence-based medicine, systematic reviews, or statistical methods to assess data. Nominators must clarify issues such as patient populations; purpose of the technology or treatment; and patient-oriented outcome parameters to be achieved. After the nomination deadline all potential topics (and their corresponding feasibility analyses) are presented to the Board of Trustees for prioritization, using a Delphi process, and final selection. The following topics were identified as priorities in 2006.

- Determination of homocysteine in blood as a risk factor for coronary disease.

- Efficacy and efficiency of drug-eluting stents compared to coronary artery bypass grafts for the treatment of coronary heart disease.

- Evaluation of stereotactic radiosurgery of meningiomas by comparison with fractionated stereotactic radiotherapy, 3D-planned conformal radiotherapy and microsurgical operations.

- Efficiency and effectiveness of behaviour-related measures for the prevention of cigarette smoking.

First, DAHTA undertakes a feasibility analysis to prioritize the topics of assessment and determine whether:

- sufficient literature is available for a topic

- the policy question needs to be conceptualized more precisely

- additional research questions need to be specified

- evaluative methods most appropriate to the question(s) have been selected.

These are investigated by systematic searches of the literature using several key databases (e.g. EMBASE, MEDLINE), and comprehensive documentation of the review process. Final assessment of the feasibility of the HTA report is based on the list of relevant literature.

Once a topic has been selected, the most suitable type of report is decided – full; methods-focused; or a brief rapid review. Moreover, assessments are either allocated in-house or commissioned from external groups. Systematic review and meta-analyses are employed as the primary methodologies for both internal and external technology assessments. When reviewing the available evidence DAHTA staff typically employ predefined protocols or guidelines, based on Cochrane Collaboration methods. Following systematic review of the evidence, the results are assembled in a draft report for review by a selected in-house committee. A final review is undertaken by the Scientific Advisory Board and HTA Board of Trustees.

DAHTA has published about 14 HTA reports since its inception in 2000, but annual numbers have been increasing. The current aim is to complete 15 reports per year. Published reports have included assessments of the value of ultrasound diagnostic techniques in the prevention of fractures; medical evaluation of using IIb/IIIa receptor blockers in the treatment of coronary syndrome patients; and a systematic overview of the methods and implementation of HTA.

IQWiG works somewhat independently from the Federal Joint Committee. It receives specific commissions for economic evaluations[56] (typically, for pharmaceutical benefit) and also is able to decide which technologies or clinical practice guidelines to assess, although there is no formal process to support these decisions. The scientific evaluation process is initiated by assembling a group of experts to define the relevant patient-outcome measures for evaluation. Therapeutic benefit must be measured against patient-relevant outcomes – typically mortality, morbidity, disease-related quality of life and convenience of use/administration. Surrogate outcome measures usually are not considered in the evaluation, as product benefit is required to be demonstrated via high-quality trials in order to qualify for reimbursement. Experts and patient organizations are consulted and supplemented by qualitative research to define the most appropriate outcome measures. A comprehensive evaluation plan is developed and published.

An evidence-based medicine approach is applied to evaluations. Typically, benefit is demonstrated by evidence from RCTs with minimal consideration of types of evidence. Most credence is given to efficacy and effectiveness data (i.e. benefit) rather than CE, but this evidence is derived from systematic synthesis of existing clinical data and literature rather than manufacturers'

---

56. However, the Institute can decide not to undertake a requested assessment if they consider that there is a lack of relevant data.

applications or submissions. Specifically, IQWiG evaluates the strength of the available evidence in relation to the:

• nature and severity of disease

• magnitude of therapeutic effect

• availability of treatment alternatives

• side-effect profile and risk of adverse events.

Experts are consulted as required during the evaluation process, especially for interpreting study results. A draft report is published for comments from stakeholders, including patients and industry. Scientific review of the quality and interpretation of the data is required and further analyses are added (see Table A5.1 for further detail). The final report summarizes and weighs the evidence of benefits and risks of the product but does not contain recommendations on reimbursement. The report is passed to the Federal Joint Committee.

HTA dissemination and implementation

The DAHTA in-house database contains all HTA publications; reports are publicly available via the web site or in book form. Moreover, HTA information is disseminated in press releases, leaflets and DIMDI newsletters, and at the annual symposia sponsored by DAHTA. DAHTA collaborates with various HTA bodies at national and international levels in order to facilitate the exposure and use of the reports, particularly the German Network for Evidence Based Medicine, the German Cochrane Centre, EUnetHTA, HTAi and ISPOR.

The Federal Joint Committee reviews the evidence provided by IQWiG to assess inclusion in the benefits catalogue and to classify the product with comparable pharmaceuticals. Reimbursement decisions are based on medical benefit followed by medical need and efficiency. The Committee defines uniform pharmaceutical reimbursement groups for agents with similar benefits and adverse effects. When the efficacy and safety of a drug is superior to existing drugs, manufacturers are able to set the price of the product for the duration of patent protection. A new drug is classified within the reference price system if it is equivalent to products already on the market. The reimbursed price for all drugs in a group is defined by the price of the cheapest product in that group.

Despite intentions in the early 2000s, price negotiations for truly innovative drugs have not been introduced. Moreover, the evaluation of drugs is not based explicitly on CE. Also, it forms the basis for inclusion in the reference pricing scheme, as described above, rather than the benefits package. There has been criticism of the use of 'jumbo groups' in the German reference pricing system. Essentially, these combine patented and non-patented drugs in a given substance class but this is considered to diminish the acknowledgement of innovative products, erode patent protection and distort the pricing structure of generic drugs.

The Federal Joint Committee's first decisions based on IQWiG evaluations were established in mid-2004 – on statins, sartans, triptans and proton pump inhibitors. Other evaluations and decisions have been made on insulin analogs and bone-marrow transplants. Since its institution, there have been a number of criticisms of IQWiG's methods. The evaluation of statins and bone-marrow transplants generated considerable debate on the appropriate use of clinical-trial data. Moreover, the unfavourable review of Exubera (claimed no advantage over existing insulin analogs) was highly criticized for not considering patient preferences on ease of use and other quality-of-life issues, despite available supporting evidence.

Broadly, IQWiG has been criticized for its methodological shortcomings – exclusion of non-trial data; lack of health economic evaluation; or not possessing a specific process for determining which technologies to assess (e.g. topics not commissioned by the Ministry). However, it is newly established and, presumably, time and experience will change its mandate and processes. Recent discussions have considered the Institute's remit and methodological approach. In the interim, some areas of the current evaluation procedures have been identified for improvement. Firstly, there appears to be a divergence between IQWiG's principal goal of quality and efficiency in health care and its evaluative methods for reaching that end. Namely, assessments neither explicitly include nor prioritize CE but rather focus narrowly on therapeutic benefit. Quality and efficiency are difficult to assess (effectively) by effects alone. Secondly, there is limited transparency about the use of stakeholders in the assessment process and the accountability of their comments and preferences in the decision-making process. Thirdly, IQWiG publishes and disseminates few assessment thereby hindering transparency and effective implementation of resulting decisions.

Table A5.1. *Overview of HTA governance, processes and role in decision-making in Germany*

Germany

HTA governance & organization

Institutions/committees	Federal Joint Committee. IGWiG. DAHTA. German Scientific Working Group of Technology Assessment in Health Care.
Entities responsible for reviewing HTA evidence for priority-setting and decision-making	Federal Joint Committee. BMG.
HTA agenda-setting body(s)	DAHTA, Federal Joint Committee/IQWiG.
Areas for HTA	IQWiG: pharmaceuticals. DAHTA: wide range of health technologies and health-care interventions/policy issues.
Reimbursement requirements and limitations	Reimbursement depends on yes/no decision for inclusion on positive list. In exceptions, conditional coverage given for particular application areas or conditions.
Stakeholder involvement	DAHTA: stakeholders can nominate assessment topics; medical and economic experts and representatives from the health-care system, patient organizations and industry participate on the leadership boards. IQWiG: experts participate on its committees; experts and patient organizations contribute to defining assessment outcome measures; stakeholders are able to comment on draft reports.
International collaboration	DAHTA: EUnetHTA, HTAi, INAHTA and ISPOR. IQWiG: G-I-N.

HTA topic selection & analytical design

Governance of topic selection	DAHTA: general public, stakeholder groups, HTA Board of Trustees.
	IQWiG: Federal Joint Committee and IQWiG.
Criteria for topic selection	DAHTA: feasibility of assessment, other criteria not stated.
Criteria for assessment	DAHTA: typically employs Cochrane Collaboration guidance to review evidence.
	IQWiG: nature and severity of disease; magnitude of therapeutic benefit; availability of treatment alternatives; side-effect profile; convenience of use.
Criteria outlined or publicly-available	By IQWiG, but not by Federal Joint Committee.
Analysis perspective	Societal.
Duration required to conduct assessments	DAHTA: average of one year.

Evidence requirements & assessment methods[57]

Documents required from manufacturer	Not relevant.
Systematic literature review and synthesis	Yes.
Unpublished data/ grey literature	Not available.
Preferred clinical study type/ evidence	RCTs.
Type of economic assessment preferred or required	Any one of cost-minimization, CE, cost-utility or cost-benefit analysis depending on the purpose of the assessment/study.

(cont.)

---

57. Section applies primarily to IQWiG.

Table A5.1. *(cont.)*

Availability of guidelines outlining methodological requirements	Yes.
Choice of comparator	Most effective form of treatment, most widely distributed or minimum practice.
Specification of outcome variable	Mortality, morbidity and quality of life.
Sub-group analyses	Not available.
Costs included in analysis	All direct and indirect costs.
Incremental analyses required	Yes.
Time horizon	Not available.
Equity issues	Not stated.
Discounting	Base case: 5% (benefits and costs); sensitivity analysis: 3%, 10% (benefits and costs).
Modelling	All inputs and assumptions must be reported and justified.
Sensitivity analyses	Analyses conducted on main uncertain parameters. Upper and lower limits must be justified.
CE or willingness-to-pay threshold	No formal threshold but likely to employ a range between €20 000 and €40 000.
Missing or incomplete data	Not available.
Support for methodological development	From DAHTA.

HTA dissemination & implementation

Channels for HTA results dissemination	DAHTA: in-house database available via web site; press releases; leaflets and DIMDI newsletters; and at the annual symposia sponsored by DAHTA.
Use of HTA results	DAHTA: primarily provides information on health-care interventions. IQWiG: supports reimbursement and pricing decisions and guideline development.
Evidence considered in decision-making	Federal Joint Committee: medical benefit, medical need and efficiency.
Any reported obstacles to effective implementation	Use of appropriate methods; narrow definition of product value/benefit (lack of incorporation of patient preferences, etc.); lack of transparency, especially for stakeholder involvement.
Formal processes to measure impact	No.
Processes for re-evaluation or appeals	IQWiG employs a review process but no formal appeals procedure.
Accountability for stakeholder input	Stakeholders involved primarily in topic identification and review of assessment reports. Not clear how stakeholder input is used in the decision-making process.
Transparent/public decision-making process	Review and accountability of Federal Joint Committee decisions undertaken by independent committees and entities, Federal Government (via the BMG) and the social courts.

Sources: Zentner et al., 2005; Busse et al., 2005; Busse & Riesberg, 2004; OECD, 2003; Perleth & Busse, 2000.

Appendix 6. United Kingdom

Overview of health-care and reimbursement systems

The United Kingdom comprises England, Scotland, Wales and Northern Ireland.[58] It is a constitutional monarchy with a principal legislative body consisting of the House of Lords and the House of Commons – the Parliament. The Prime Minister appoints a cabinet of senior ministers, most of whom head the main departments of state. These secretaries of state and other ministers account to Parliament for the work of their departments, including major policy initiatives and decisions.

Responsibility for health and personal social services in England lies with the Department of Health (DH), under the auspices of the Secretary of State for Health and associated ministerial bodies.[59] Separate responsibilities are held by the Secretaries of State for Scotland, Wales and Northern Ireland respectively. In England, the DH sets overall health policy (including policies on public health, the environment and food matters) and has responsibility for the National Health Service (NHS). In practice, health and health service provision and policy are broadly similar across the United Kingdom (Woolf & Henshall, 2000), although there has been some divergence since the founding of the Scottish Parliament.

The NHS was created under the National Health Services Act 1946 to provide universal health coverage for all citizens. It is financed mainly through central government taxation, with an element of national insurance contributions. Most services are free of charge at the time of delivery, although modest co-payments apply to some medicines, dental services and eye care.

Several core principles underpin the NHS Directive (Department of Health, 2000).

• Provision of services based on need rather than ability to pay.

• Provision of a comprehensive range of services.

• Services will be developed around the individual needs of patients and different patient populations.

• Services will be of high quality and with minimal errors.

• Public funds for health care will be dedicated solely to NHS patients.

---

58. This case study focuses on England and Wales.

59. Includes Ministries of Social Security; Environment, Transport and the Regions; Agriculture, Food and Fisheries; and the Department of Education and Employment.

- NHS will strive to protect the health of individuals and reduce health inequalities.

- NHS will respect individual confidentiality and will provide open access to information about services, treatment and performance.

Care provision is grounded in fairness and consistency; the availability of services is determined by effectiveness (clinically appropriate) and CE (Department of Health, 1997). To that end, the NHS is not obliged to provide specified services, only those "necessary to meet reasonable requirements."[60] The Secretary of State is able to take account of economic factors, specifically NHS financial capacity, but blanket bans on particular services are prohibited (Mason & Smith, 2005).[61] Within the NHS there are no specific entitlements to services, but little is explicitly excluded.

Primary Care Trusts (PCTs) and Strategic Health Authorities (SHAs) have the mandate to ensure that the establishment and delivery of NHS services meets requirements and standards.[62] More specifically, SHAs promote comprehensive services while PCTs are responsible for prioritizing service provision within their respective financial budgets. Legislation requires these entities to regard the principles of the NHS Directive when exercising their functions.

To complement its core principles and to meet "reasonable requirements", the NHS Plan of 2000 emphasized the role of implementation and delivery, focusing on components such as the national service frameworks (NSFs); NICE; waiting-time guarantees; and guidance from the DH (Mason & Smith, 2005). These measures also help to specify the conditions under which patients may be eligible for health-care services. Taken together, these mechanisms contribute to regulatory quality and control, and protect rights to health care. The Healthcare Commission is responsible for monitoring compliance among NHS organizations and regulating adherence to these standards.

Introduced in the 1997 White Paper, NSFs aim to improve quality and reduce variations in services by introducing standards, identifying key interventions for particular patient group(s) and establishing strategies to

---

60. This partly explains the variations in local service provision known as the post-code lottery.

61. However, exceptions are made for treatments with overwhelming evidence of clinical ineffectiveness. Exclusions typically cover medicines and screening.

62. PCTs are responsible for managing local primary health-care services and control approximately 80% of the NHS budget. SHAs are responsible for developing plans for improving local health services; monitoring quality and performance; managing the capacity of health-care services; and ensuring that national priorities are integrated into local health plans. Essentially, SHAs provide a key link between the DH and the NHS. As of July 2006, there were approximately 10 SHAs.

facilitate implementation. Essentially, NSFs serve as positive guidance and do not explicitly proscribe interventions (Mason & Smith, 2005). To date, they have addressed a wide range of topics including cancer, diabetes and long-term conditions. For coronary heart disease, the NSF set 12 standards for improved prevention, diagnosis and treatment; and goals to secure equitable access to high-quality services. Typically, one NSF is produced every year (Mason & Smith, 2005).

Introduced in 1999, NICE was created to promote clinical excellence within the NHS by reducing variation in the uptake of new health technologies (Newdick, 2005). Part of its remit is to support the effective use of resources and include CE in decisions. NICE produces three types of guidance: technology appraisals, clinical guidelines and interventional procedures. Since mid-2005, it has assumed the Health Development Agency's responsibilities for evaluating public health interventions.

NICE guidance serves a quasi-legal function, but one aspect of technology appraisals is supported by mandate. Associated health-care organizations are obliged to implement NICE recommendations for a particular technology to be available to certain patient group(s) (Mason & Smith, 2005). Moreover, they are required to do so within three months of the guidance's publication date (see *HTA procedures and processes* below).

The DH also often develops and disseminates guidance on a range of health-care issues. Typically, the principal form of guidance is health service circulars (HSCs) that frequently supplement local authority circulars (LACs). Although these circulars generally call for a specific quasi-legislative action, some take the form of directives from the Secretary of Health and, therefore, are legally-binding. Guidance is also generated specifically for the PCTs and other Trusts, typically promulgated by the SHAs.

Beyond NICE, several arms-length entities service the NHS under four broad areas: regulation, standards, public welfare and central services (Mason & Smith, 2005). The key bodies are described below.

- *Healthcare Commission.* Independent regulatory body for NHS and private health-care organizations. Regulatory activity assesses compliance with DH-set standards to ensure quality of care and organizations' capacity to deliver these services to patients. Health-care organizations are evaluated according to adherence to standards related to safety; clinical- and cost-effectiveness; governance; patient focus; accessible and responsible care; amenities and care environment; and public health.

- *Monitor.* Independent public body that promotes comprehensive health services; provides facilities to medical and dental schools; and ensures financial sustainability of NHS Foundation Trusts.[63] Stipulates the goods and services that may be provided by Foundation Trusts.

- *Medicines and Healthcare products Regulatory Agency (MHRA).* Executive agency of the DH responsible for ensuring that medicines and other medical products meet appropriate standards of quality, safety, performance, effectiveness and appropriate use. As part of its remit assesses the safety, quality and efficacy of medicines; authorizes medicines; operates post-market surveillance monitoring; regulates clinical trials; evaluates regulatory compliance via inspection; and promotes safe use of medicines.

- *Pharmaceutical Price Regulation Scheme (PPRS).* Seeks to secure the provision of safe and effective medicines at responsible prices; promote competition within the pharmaceutical industry; and support the development and supply of medicines. Embodies a series of rules focused on regulating pharmaceutical companies' profits from medicine sales to the NHS. Impacts on CE by influencing companies' decisions about the prices of individual medicines in the United Kingdom.

Several other entities play key roles in the British health system, including consumer and voluntary groups, professional bodies (e.g. British Medical Association) and the private sector. Private health insurers act primarily as a safety net for cases where demand exceeds NHS supply, with patients relying either on insurance coverage or self-payments.

HTA governance and organization

As in most countries, the rapid emergence of new and expensive health technologies is a major contributing factor to rising heath-care costs. Some estimates have indicated that technological advances cause NHS costs to increase by an average of 0.5% to 1% per year (Woolf & Henshall, 2000). Rising costs and resource-limited health-care budgets have resulted in a growing emphasis on priority-setting and focusing resources on interventions that offer patients effective and affordable benefits. Moreover, evidence regarding effectiveness (and CE) increasingly has been a focus of NHS programmes.

In this context, HTA has emerged as a policy priority in the United Kingdom, not only to determine the most appropriate interventions for health-care services, but also to improve the quality and value of allocated resources.

---

63. Foundation Trusts are a new type of NHS organization aimed at decentralizing health-care decision-making and service provision. Firmly situated within the NHS and abiding by NHS standards, they are accountable to local communities rather than central government.

Consequently, there has been widespread activity in HTA in recent years. Much has stemmed from the DH, NICE and the NCCHTA but there is on-going activity in various entities throughout the United Kingdom, not restricted to NHS programmes.

NICE is an independent organization responsible for providing national guidance on a variety of health interventions. Specifically, its roles and responsibilities include the production of guidance on public health, health technologies and clinical practice. NICE guidance for public health focuses solely on England; guidance on health technologies and clinical practice covers England and Wales; guidance on interventional procedures covers England, Wales and Scotland.

NICE is structured across three different centres – the Centre for Public Health Excellence, Centre for Health Technology Evaluation and the Centre for Clinical Practice. Created in April 2005, the Centre for Public Health Excellence develops guidance on topics central to public *Health Policy* (the promotion of good health and disease prevention) targeted towards practitioners and policy-makers in the NHS; local authorities; private and voluntary sectors; and the general public.

The Centre for Public Health Excellence is organized into three Public Health Programme Development Groups (PDGs). These comprise researchers and practitioners; representatives of the stakeholders of the topic under evaluation; and individuals supporting the general public, as appropriate. Each is headed by an Associate Centre Director who is a leader in the public health field. PDGs are responsible for supporting the development of public health guidance by scoping topics, engaging with stakeholders, organizing reviews of the guidance and managing public consultation (NICE, 2006a). They devise final recommendations following consultation. The directors support and direct the respective groups on generating evidence and developing guidance; and manage any work with collaborating centres.

On a more general level, the Public Health Interventions Advisory Committee (PHIAC) reviews the guidance developed by the PDGs (NICE, 2006a) and comprises health researchers, statisticians, epidemiologists, methodologists, practitioners and lay stakeholder groups. It is assisted by specialist advisers – clinicians nominated or approved by professional bodies. In some cases, specialists in a particular subject are invited to provide expert testimony by participating in committee meetings. Moreover, NICE has commissioned a review body, composed of universities and a teaching hospital, to provide systematic reviews of interventional procedures and collect data.

The Centre for Health Technology Evaluation develops guidance on the use of new and existing medicines, treatments and procedures within the NHS.

Its work is overseen by three primary entities: the Interventional Procedure Advisory Committee (IPAC), independent academic centres and the Technology Appraisal Committee. The IPAC includes NHS heath professionals and others familiar with key issues affecting patients. It also collaborates with specialist advisers nominated by relevant health professional bodies.

The Centre often commissions an independent academic centre to prepare technology assessment reports (TARs) for consideration by the Technology Appraisal Committee (see below). In particular, NICE collaborates with the following TAR teams or centres (NICE, 2004a).

- Health Economics Research Unit and Health Services Research Unit, University of Aberdeen;

- Liverpool Reviews and Implementation Group, University of Liverpool;

- Centre for Reviews and Dissemination and Centre for Health Economics, University of York;

- Peninsula Technology Assessment Group (PenTAG), Peninsula Medical School, Universities of Exeter and Plymouth;

- School of Health and Related Research (ScHARR), University of Sheffield;

- Southampton Health Technology Assessments Centre (SHTAC), University of Southampton;

- West Midlands Health Technology Assessment Collaboration, Department of Public Health and Epidemiology, University of Birmingham.

Although part of the Centre for Health Technology Evaluation, the Technology Appraisal Committee is an independent entity with membership drawn from the NHS, patient organizations, academia and industry. Members typically are appointed for a three-year term and allocated to one of two branches within the Committee (NICE, 2004a).

The Centre for Health Technology Evaluation also confers with various consultee organizations ranging from national patient groups, health professional bodies and manufacturers of the technology under review. Such entities are able to submit evidence during the evaluation process, comment on appraisal documents and appeal against the Appraisal Committee's final recommendations. Commentator organizations are represented by manufacturers of comparator products, NHS Quality Improvement Scotland (QIS) and research groups working in the relevant topic areas. These bodies can comment on evidence and other documents used or produced by the appraisal process, but cannot submit evidence.

The Centre for Clinical Practice offers guidance on the appropriate treatment of specific diseases and conditions within the NHS. The guidelines interpret and provide guidance on how to implement the NSFs. Representatives from the Medical Royal Colleges, professional bodies and patient organizations form national collaborating centres (NCCs) to help to manage guideline development and publication. The seven NCCs oversee different disease areas such as cancer, mental health and chronic conditions. Guidelines are developed by establishing a Guideline Development Group comprising members with expertise in systematic review; evidence appraisal; clinical- and cost-effectiveness; and patient issues. Registered stakeholders are invited to nominate members. The Guideline Development Group also consults with stakeholders to inform guideline development.

The Centre for Clinical Practice also has a number of Guideline Review Panels, typically consisting of four or five members (including chairperson and deputy), which serve to validate the final complete guidelines. In particular, they focus on how comments received during the consultation process were considered in the final guideline.

NICE also houses a board, with various sub-committees and partner and citizens' councils. The Citizens Council assists NICE's decision-making and informs the development of guidance by providing general public opinions on key issues. This council consists of approximately 30 individuals drawn from various population groups. Participation is open to the broader public and its value lies in involvement from stakeholders that typically are not represented in the assessment process. For this reason NHS employees, patient groups and representatives of lobbying organizations and industry are not allowed to participate (NICE, 2004b). Independent facilitators (with no direct association to NICE) recruit members.

Collaboration between NICE's various centres is encouraged and increasingly commonplace. For example, the outputs of one centre may be used in guidance produced by other bodies (e.g. technology appraisals often inform clinical guidance). This coordination allows for a more coherent presentation of advice to stakeholders and efficient use of resource and expertise within the Institute.

Part of the Wessex Institute for Health Research and Development at the University of Southampton, the NCCHTA is another primary HTA body in the United Kingdom. This manages, supports and develops the NHS HTA programme on behalf of the DH Research and Development Division. The NHS HTA programme provides information on the costs, effectiveness and broader impacts of health technologies specifically for those who use, manage and provide care in the NHS. Additionally, it supports NICE by managing

TAR contracts and contributing to STAs (see HTA processes and procedures), and by commissioning Evidence Review Group reports which appraise manufacturers' submissions.

Research activities within the NCCHTA rely on a number of different internal and external expert bodies. Various experts contribute as members of HTA panels, the HTA Expert Advisory Network, the Prioritization Strategy Group, the HTA Commissioning Board and the HTA Clinical Trials Board. Individual experts and referees provide input on research proposals and final reports. The HTA panels' key function is to set research priorities within four different areas: pharmaceuticals; diagnostic technologies and screening; therapeutic procedures; and disease prevention. The HTA Expert Advisory Network provides HTA panels with a comprehensive range of expertise on care topics and settings, thereby supplementing the specialties and disciplines provided by other entities. The Prioritization Strategy Group was established to develop an HTA research portfolio according to the needs of the NHS and available research with the HTA programme budget. The HTA Commissioning Board is principally responsible for assessing prioritized research proposals but also makes funding recommendations to the HTA programme director, typically two or three times per year. The HTA Clinical Trials Board considers research proposals for clinical trials to assess the effectiveness of technologies within the NHS.

In addition to formalized committees, the NCCHTA actively involves the public in the assessment process through some level of participation in (NCCHTA, 2006):

- identifying topics for research

- reviewing and prioritizing research proposals

- reviewing draft assessment reports

- agenda-setting for R&D priorities in the NHS and future public involvement.

A number of other entities engage in HTA activities across the United Kingdom. These include the commercial and charitable sectors, academia, Medical Research Council, National Horizon Scanning Centre, the UK Cochrane Centre and the Committee on the Safety of Medicines and Joint Committee Vaccination and Immunisation. In addition, NHS Trusts produce their own local formularies and often have committees to assess the impact of new medicines on their own budgets and on primary care.

HTA process and procedures[64]

The guideline development process is initiated when NICE receives suggestions for topics from a number of sources. In general, the DH commissions NICE to develop clinical guidelines, guidance on public health and technology appraisals. Topics for the interventional procedures programme are submitted directly to NICE, usually by clinicians. Other topics for potential NICE guidance are submitted by public heath professionals, patients and the general public; the National Horizon Scanning Centre; and internally. Public health professionals, patients and the general public submit suggested topics via on-line or hard-copy forms. Manufacturers submit topic requests to the National Horizon Scanning Centre, which informs the DH about key new and emerging technologies that might require NICE evaluations.

After a public consultation process in mid-2006 NICE became responsible for the initial stages of the topic selection process, on behalf of the DH. A submitted topic is reviewed for appropriateness[65] and then filtered according to several DH criteria. The list of selection criteria was created in July 2006, following a public consultation process and includes (NICE, 2006b):

• burden of disease (population affected, morbidity, mortality);

• resource impact (cost impact on the NHS or the public sector);

• clinical and policy importance (whether topic falls within a government priority area);

• presence of inappropriate variation(s) in practice;

• potential factors affecting the timeliness of the proposed guidance (degree of urgency, relevancy at the expected date of delivery);

• likelihood of guidance having an impact on public health and quality of life, the reduction of health inequalities, or the delivery of quality programmes or interventions.

A panel composed of experts in the relevant topic area, generalists with a substantial knowledge of health services and delivery, public health professionals, and patient representatives review the topic suggestions according to these criteria. Their recommendations are reviewed by ministers at the DH who have final responsibility for selecting the topics referred to NICE for guidance development.

---

64. Section focuses on NICE HTA processes and procedures.

65. Appropriateness measured by whether topic is within NICE's remit; NICE has already produced or developed guidance on the topic; topic represents an emerging public health issue; topic is an ultra-orphan disease.

NICE employs slightly different assessment processes depending on the type of guidance. Two types of guidance are produced for public health issues – public health intervention and programme guidance. The process for public health intervention guidance follows the steps below (NICE, 2006a).

Topic selection

See above.

Registration of stakeholders

Those with an interest in participating in the guidance development process (e.g. professional organizations, research and academic institutions, industry, general public) are requested to register with NICE.

Preparation of project scope

Outline of guidance content and development process is prepared and, following a consultation process, finalized. This aims to:

- provide clear definition of the topic;

- identify relevant care settings, health delivery systems and providers;

- ascertain policy context; develop key questions (related to effectiveness, CE, feasibility and acceptability, among other factors);

- establish clear timelines;

- specify outcome measures and any comparators.

An initial literature search and the development of a conceptual and analytical framework help to inform and guide preparation of the scope.

Systematic review of evidence

NICE or an external research body conducts a review of evidence and economic appraisal of the public health intervention. The review synopsis is disseminated to registered stakeholders for comment.

Reviews are based on the best available evidence drawn from a range of disciplines and research traditions. Evidence is selected and appraised according to well-defined criteria, based on their appropriateness for answering the research questions. NICE requires the process for identifying the evidence to be as transparent as possible; all search strategies and terms must be documented. Typically, each review will use one or more of the following sources of evidence:

- evidence briefing (review of reviews)

- systematic review of primary data

- existing, published primary research

- new primary research, where appropriate and if time and resources allow.

Stakeholders are also invited to submit potential evidence (e.g. systematic reviews, RCTs, epidemiological studies, other guidelines on the topic, economic models, etc.) during consultations on the synopsis.

The review process involves a number of standardized steps – assessing the quality of the selected evidence; extracting and synthesizing (e.g. evidence tables, meta-analyses); and developing the evidence statement (summary for each of the key questions). The economic component of the appraisal is typically conducted if the topic is deemed a priority area. This is measured by:

- presence of major resource implications

- potential challenges to current public health practice

- data sufficient for modelling

- lack of consensus among public health professionals.

Usually, a systematic review of the evidence is undertaken based on a standardized guidance document outlining steps for reviewing evidence, documenting the quality of studies, etc. Moreover, reviewers follow a methodology checklist in the economic evaluation. Further information on the methods used in the economic evaluation is detailed in Table A6.2.

Whichever analytical approach is used, all economic evaluation is underpinned by transparency in the reporting of methods and any uncertainty about internal and external validity. Moreover, the limitations of the methods used are discussed fully.

Drafting of the guidance

PHIAC reviews the synopsis and drafts the guidance. Recommendations are based on several factors including the strength of supporting evidence, importance of outcomes, health impact, CE and other considerations (e.g. inequalities, implementation/feasibility).

Consultation

The draft guidance undergoes a one-month consultation period.

Conduct of fieldwork

The draft guidance is tested via meetings with practitioners in the field. Meeting reports are drafted in a technical document and submitted to PHIAC.

Field meetings are predicated on the notion that successful implementation of guidance depends on evidence-based recommendations informed by practical experience. To meet this end, at least four to five full-day meetings are convened across a variety of geographical regions. Independent professional facilitators are present for each meeting to which, typically, a maximum of 35 practitioners (with experience related to the topic) is invited. The series of meetings covers the work environment in which the practitioners operate, evidence reviewed during the assessment and the subsequent draft guideline and recommendations. All meetings are recorded to ensure transparency and accuracy of information.

Production of the final guidance

PHIAC produces the final guidance having reviewed the technical document and comments from the consultation period.

Approval and issue of guideline

Following peer review, NICE formally approves the final guidance and disseminates it to the NHS.

The development procedure for programme guidance is similar, except that a Programme Development Group (PDG) is created to draft and finalize the guidance (responsibilities similar to the Advisory Committee).

The assessment process for interventional procedures' guidance entails the following steps (NICE, 2004g).

Notification of procedures

Typically, physicians notify NICE of potential procedures for review but all stakeholders may submit a request. The National Horizon Scanning Centre is a stakeholder that notifies NICE of procedures likely to be used for the first time within the next year. NICE primarily investigates new procedures and compiles and maintains a list of all notified procedures.

Registration of stakeholders

See section on public health intervention guidance.

Preparation of overview

An overview of the procedure is prepared in collaboration with at least three specialist advisers. This summarizes the nature and purpose of the procedure; results of valid studies found in a rapid literature review; key safety and efficacy issues; and opinions of the specialist advisers. Overview documents are not the result of a systematic review.

Device manufacturers and other stakeholders can submit or alert NICE to any new evidence or publications relevant to the procedure. Other non-confidential information may also be submitted at this stage.

Referral to the review body

IPAC reviews the overview document for public health impact, innovation of the procedure, adverse event profile and potential uptake. This forms the basis of the decision to refer the procedure to the review body for further investigation that typically involves a systematic review and/or collection and analysis of data.

Production of consultation document

The review body's report informs the decision on whether to continue with the process or to collect additional data. The process continues with the production of a consultation document that outlines the safety and efficacy associated with the procedure using evidence from the review body. The document and all supporting materials (e.g. technology appraisals, guidelines) are posted on the NICE web site for comment (open for 4 weeks) and key stakeholders are notified.

Development of final recommendations

Following the consultation period, IPAC considers the efficacy and safety of the procedure. Such considerations may or may not involve comparison with other procedures or treatments. Final recommendations are submitted to NICE for approval.

Notification of recommendations

Following approval, consultees (see HTA governance and organization) are requested to review the guidance. Those who feel that the guidance is inaccurate, or have a complaint with the development process, can submit a resolution within 15 days.

Issuance of guidance

Guidance is issued to the NHS. Cases with sufficient evidence of a procedure's safety and efficacy may be referred to the Advisory Committee on Topic Selection and recommended for a technology appraisal.

NICE not only publishes the consultation document and the final guidance on the web site, but also publishes the overview summary, minutes of advisory committee meetings, reports from the review body and any evidence pivotal to the committees' decisions, with the exception of unpublished data deemed "commercial or academic in confidence". This ensures transparency of the guidance development process.

NICE produces three different versions of technology appraisals: full appraisals, quick reference guides and information for the public. Each version targets different stakeholder groups, from the NHS and health professionals (full appraisals and quick reference guides) to patient groups and a lay audience (information for the public).

The process for technology appraisals is similar to that used for developing public health guidance and is outlined below (NICE, 2004a, NICE, 2004c, NICE, 2004f).

Provisional list of appraisal topics

The DH produces a list of provisional appraisal topics.

Identification of consultees and commentators

Preparation of project scope (see above also)

However, NICE develops the scope for technology appraisals through collaboration with the DH. Unless the DH specifies otherwise, appraisals do not normally consider the use of technology for indications which have not been granted regulatory approval in the United Kingdom.

A consultation process with the consultees and commentators is initiated for each potential appraisal topic. The scope is reviewed and made available for comment. Manufacturers' comments are required to include any information on pending licence applications and the time frame for regulatory approval. The draft scope is also posted on the NICE web site.

NICE convenes a scoping workshop with consultees and commentators, the DH and the Welsh Assembly Government. Amendments are made where necessary. The finalized scope is submitted to the Ministers of

Health who decide whether the technology appraisal is suitable for formal referral to NICE (see above for more information on topic selection).

Preparation of the appraisal

The assessment group (typically one of the TAC groups) is formally commissioned (in conference between NICE and the NHS HTA Programme, through the NCCHTA) to prepare the report upon issuance of the final scope and list of consultees and commentators. These are published together with the timelines on the NICE web site.

Manufacturers are asked to prepare a written submission containing available evidence on clinical- and cost-effectiveness. This is sent to the assessment group and used to inform the assessment report. The transparency of the appraisal process is upheld by all evidence pivotal to the Committee's decision being made publicly available. Under particular circumstances, NICE accepts unpublished or part-published evidence under an agreement of confidentiality. This is particularly true for technologies undergoing appraisal immediately prior to regulatory approval that includes commercial and/or academic in confidence data. At a minimum, a structured abstract should be made available for public disclosure. All confidential information is available for review by the assessment group and appraisal Committee. The same principles apply to the release of information submitted via economic models – they must be included with the written submission in electronic format.

Manufacturers are required to identify all studies relevant to the appraisal in the form of clinical trials, follow-up studies and registry evidence. Cohort studies and case series require a full report of baseline characteristics, the rationale for case selection and the best equivalent evidence on the best available treatment for patients. Moreover, manufacturers are asked to comment on any other factors to be taken into account when interpreting clinical- and cost-effectiveness.

Development of the assessment report

The assessment group reviews the clinical and cost-effectiveness of the technology based on a systematic review of the literature and manufacturers' submissions to NICE. The evidence of therapeutic effect considered in the review ranges from RCTs to observational studies, although head-to-head clinical trials are preferred. Evidence requirements for CE include benefit on the course of disease; impact on patients' health-related quality of life; and the value of those impacts in representation of patient preferences. Also, evidence of the technology's effect on resource use and its valuation in monetary terms. Evidence of CE can be obtained from original analyses and/or systematic reviews of existing published literature. Evidence on acceptability, appropriateness, preference, feasibility and equity are also considered where relevant and available.

Evidence typically is submitted by the assessment group, manufacturers, patient groups and health professionals/providers. The assessment group also gathers evidence from consultations with clinical and methodological experts and may produce an economic model in support of the report. These models are owned by the relevant assessment group and cannot be used for any purpose other than informing the assessment. Further details on the methods used for assembling and synthesizing evidence to estimate the clinical- and cost-effectiveness of the technology being appraised are provided in Table A6.2.

Assessment reports are not comprehensive reviews of all the information on a given technology. Rather they are focused assessments of the evidence pertinent to the defined scopes. Assessment groups use submitted evidence according to how closely it aligns with the criteria defined in the assessment protocols and follows recognized methodological guidance.

Typically, reports are allocated a time frame of approximately 36 weeks. A completed report is submitted to NICE to form the basis of an appraisal. NICE instructs the consultees and commentators that the report is available for comment.

Development of the evaluation report

The assessment report and other evidence and comments from consultees and commentators are combined into an evaluation report. This does not propose recommendations on the use of the technology, but develops recommendations that form the guidance on the use of the technology within the NHS.

Production of the appraisal consultation document (ACD)

The evaluation report is submitted to an independent appraisal committee. Nominated clinical specialists and patient experts participate in the committee meeting at which they can respond to and pose questions. The ACD contains the committee's recommendations on a treatment's clinical- and cost-effectiveness for use within the NHS. It may recommend against the use of treatment where the benefits to patients are unproven or not cost-effective but is not responsible for making recommendations on the pricing of the technologies to the NHS.

The following factors are considered during the appraisal:

• nature and quality of the evidence;

• uncertainty generated by the evidence and difference between the evidence submitted for licensing and that related to effectiveness in clinical practice;

• consideration of effectiveness and adverse events in different subgroups of patients;

• risks and benefits of the technology from the patient's perspective;

• position of the technology in the overall care pathway and in relation to alternative treatments;

• implications for health-care programmes from adoption of the new technology;

• appropriateness of the comparator technology(s), as perceived by NHS stakeholders;

• estimates of CE (as evidenced by the incremental CE ratio);[66]

• robustness of the economic methods (e.g. modelling, sensitivity analysis);

• broad clinical and policy government priorities;

• extent of health need;

• effective use of available resources;

• long-term objective of encouraging innovation that will benefit NHS patients.

The ACD highlights the key evidence used in the appraisal process and any areas of contention or uncertainty. The finalized document is made available to the consultees and commentators, health professionals and the public. Comments are requested over a four-week period.

If new data that materially impact the ACD's provisional recommendations become available during the appraisal process, the appraisal committee may choose to re-formulate it for additional rounds of consultation.

---

66. NICE does not apply a fixed willingness-to-pay threshold, but bases decisions primarily on the CE estimate for incremental CE ratios below £ 20 000 per QALY (Rawlins & Culyer, 2004). However, as the incremental CE ratio increases, the likelihood of rejection on the grounds of cost-ineffectiveness rises. Typically, NICE requires additional justification for ratios over £ 25 000 per QALY. Particular considerations would include the degree of uncertainty surrounding the estimate; equity and public health impacts; and the innovative nature of the technology.

Such data would typically include new trial data, new analysis or modification of the economic model and changes in the licensed indications of the technology.

Production of the final appraisal determination (FAD)

The appraisal committee reviews the comments on the ACD. Its final recommendations are published in the FAD and submitted to NICE for final approval. The process takes approximately 14 weeks.

Consultees may appeal against the FAD or the way in which the appraisal process was conducted. The grounds for appeal include:

- NICE has failed to act in accordance with its published appraisal procedures

- FAD does not reflect submitted evidence

- NICE has exceeded its remit.

At the discretion of the appeal committee, appellants are given an opportunity to make an oral submission of complaint.

Issue of guidance

If there are no appeals or none is upheld, NICE officially issues the guidance (technical appraisal guidance – TAG).

NICE facilitates the transparency of the appraisal process by making the majority of evidence pivotal to decision-making publicly available, with the exception of commercial and academic in confidence data.

In addition to the appraisal procedure (multiple technology appraisal – MTA) described, in 2005 NICE developed a process for the appraisal of single technologies for a sole indication (single technology appraisal – STA). These are used for new pharmaceutical products close to market launch; cases where most relevant evidence lies with the manufacturer or sponsor. The decision on the appropriateness of the STA process is made during the topic selection stage (see above). Typically, selection is based on factors such as the complexity of current standard treatments and the likelihood of the main evidence base being held by the sponsor. The STA process is used to ensure that NICE is able to issue prompt guidance to the NHS when new technology is introduced into the United Kingdom market.

The STA process is similar to that of the full appraisal process described, but only the manufacturer's evidence submission is considered formally in the independent review. Moreover, formal consultation procedures take place only if the appraisal committee's preliminary recommendations are substantially more restrictive than the terms of the licence indication under appraisal (NICE, 2006c). The STA process has different timelines too (NICE, 2006c). Specifically, less time is required to produce the guidance: approximately 32 to 39 weeks from initiation of the appraisal to publication. The FAD is made publicly available at 27 and 35 weeks. Where the appraisal tracks regulatory approval the first appraisal committee meeting is organized following a positive opinion from EMEA. The minimum time from regulatory approval to publication of the guidance is between 6 and 13 weeks.

STA guidance is considered for review following publication. The time between publication and review varies according to the anticipated rate of development of evidence for the technology and prior knowledge of the completion of pivotal research (NICE, 2006c). In general, this period spans one to five years. To date, the STA process has been applied to drugs, mainly those for cancer.

Lastly, NICE produces clinical guidelines aimed at improving the quality of health care by providing recommendations for treatment and informing standards for health-care professionals and decision-making among patients. NICE develops four versions: full guideline, NICE guideline, quick reference guide and information for the public.

The guideline-development process is similar to that for public health interventions and described briefly below (NICE, 2006d, NICE, 2006e).

Topic selection

See above.

Registration of stakeholders

Preparation of project scope and work plan

The NCC commissioned to develop the guideline prepares the scope in collaboration with NICE, registered stakeholders and an independent guideline review panel (see previous sections for further details). An initial literature search and development of a conceptual and analytical framework inform and guide preparation of the scope.

The scope is subject to consultation with stakeholders over a four-week period, during which the scope is published on the NICE web site. NICE approves the scope following a review and responses to any comments.

A work plan is devised to specify methods, timelines and cost. This forms an agreement for NICE and the NCC to develop the guideline.

Establish guideline development group

These groups comprise health professionals, representatives of patient organizations and technical experts. Registered stakeholders can nominate participants.

Systematic review of evidence

Evidence that supports the guidance typically is derived from searches of electronic databases and via information submitted by stakeholder organizations (see section on public health intervention guidance).

A health economist participates in the guideline development group to advise on economic issues, review the economic literature and recommend components of the review or guideline that would benefit from original economic analysis, such as CE analyses or modelling. Table A6.2 outlines the methods used in the guideline development process.

If there is insufficient evidence to reach consensus on the recommendations, focus groups and/or a formal consensus process (e.g. Delphi panels) are pursued.

Drafting of the guideline

The guideline development group prioritizes guideline recommendations by:

- impact on patient outcomes
- impact on reducing variations in practice
- ability to lead to more efficient use of NHS resources
- expediency of patient movement through the care pathway.

Moreover, recommendations typically involve areas that require further research in order to inform a guideline update.

Consultation on the draft guidance

There is a minimum of one consultation period for registered stakeholders to comment on the draft guideline. Following the consultation period(s), the guideline review panel ensures that stakeholder comments are considered, where appropriate.

Production of the final guidance

The review panel finalizes the recommendations and sends the draft guidance to the NCC for production of the final guideline.

Approval and issue of guideline

NICE formally approves the final guidance and disseminates it to the NHS.

In addition to this clinical guideline process, NICE has recently instituted short clinical guidelines. These are designed to address clinical questions that do not meet the criteria for a traditional clinical guideline or technology appraisal, but would benefit from more urgent guidance. The short guideline is developed in the same manner, but within a shorter timescale, typically between 9 to 11 months.

Table A6.1 details examples of published and planned NICE guidance over the last five years. To date, NICE has completed approximately 90 appraisals (Cairns, 2006).

HTA dissemination and implementation

The guidelines and guidance produced by NICE are employed on a number of different levels. They have been used to:

- develop treatment standards for health organizations;

- inform and guide decision-making among patients and consumers;

- guide actions to meet government indicators and targets for health improvement and to reduce health inequalities;

- improve communication between patients and providers;

- guide education and training of health professionals;

- reduce variations in treatment and practice;

- inform decision-making on NHS funding and resource allocation;

- guide the development of treatment pathways for new procedures and interventions.

To facilitate dissemination, all publications focus on the needs of different stakeholder groups – government and NHS decision-makers, health professionals, patients and the general public. All guidance is published online and NICE also send copies to NHS chief executives; local government organizations; health professionals working in areas covered by the guidance; NHS staff responsible for clinical governance; consultants in relevant specialties; medical, nursing and public health directors of NHS Boards and Trusts; and the Healthcare Commission, among many others. Moreover, NICE informs the broadcast and print media about newly published guidance and participates in various HTA international organizations and professional societies such as HTAi.

The Secretary of State has instituted a mandatory requirement that Health Commissioners make funds available for implementation of guidances

Table A6.1. *Examples of published and planned NICE guidance*

Public health guidance		Interventional procedures guidance		Technology appraisals		Clinical guidelines	
Published	Planned	Published	Planned	Published	Planned	Published	Planned
Physical activity	Alcohol & schools intervention	Deep brain stimulation for tremor and dystonia	Transcranial magnetic stimulation for severe depression	Bipolar disorder – new drugs	Asthma (uncontrolled) – omalizumab	Hypertension	Breast cancer
Smoking cessation	Mental health & older people	Insertion of biological slings for stress urinary incontinence	Arthroscopic knee washout	Crohn's disease – infliximab	Hearing impairment – cochlear implants	Caesarean section	Low back pain
	Substance misuse	Laparoscopic partial nephrectomy	Cryotherapy for renal cancers	Obesity – orlistat	Pulmonary arterial hypertension – drugs	Lung cancer	Incontinence
	Preventing STDs and pregnancy in those under 18	High-intensity focused ultrasound for prostate cancer		Sepsis (severe) – drotrecogin	Drug misuse – naltrexone	Self-harm	Obesity
	Workplace smoking					Urinary incontinence	Stroke

produced from technology appraisals, within three months of publication. QIS reviews published NICE guidance for its implications and validity for adoption by NHS Scotland. However, the NHS Boards in Scotland are not obliged to provide funds for the implementation of NICE guidance.

NICE has established a programme to aid the implementation of guidance (including technology appraisals). Each guidance is assigned an implementation team that collaborates with those involved in the development process. Communications and field-based teams ensure targeted dissemination to various audiences; engage with the NHS, local government and the wider community; evaluate uptake; and raise awareness of NICE guidance.

Moreover, NICE provides a number of tools to support the implementation of guidance, all available via the web site (NICE, 2006f).

- Forward planner – summarizes published and forthcoming NICE guidance; explains which sectors are likely to be impacted.

- Slide sets – highlight key messages from the guidance and make recommendations for implementation.

- Audit criteria – assist organizations to execute baseline assessment and monitor associated activities.

- Costing tools – help to assess the financial impact of implementing NICE guidance.

- Implementation advice – points to sources of support, resources, etc.

- Commissioning guides – provide support for local commissioning and needs assessment.

- Evaluation and review of NICE implementation evidence (ERNIE) database – provides details on how NICE guidance is being used.

NICE also tracks the implementation of its guidance within NHS Trusts. Appraisals are re-evaluated every four years for health technologies; every four to six years for clinical guidelines; every three years for public health guidance; and every one to five years for STAs. As described, NICE incorporates a formal appeals process for each type of guidance. There have been about 20 appeals to date.

Overall, NICE and its programmes for developing guidance are unique and represent a policy embodiment of evidence-based medicine. Culyer (2006) describes how NICE promulgates a deliberate process that elicits and combines various types of evidence from different sources in order to develop guidance. Several aspects inherent to NICE's procedures produce an effective deliberative process, many focus on ensuring the highest degree of transparency and the participation of a wide range of stakeholders. Such characteristics include:

- bi-monthly open board meetings across England and Wales;

- broadly set membership of the technology appraisal committee;

- existence of, and participation in, partners and citizens councils;

- extensive consultation and comment opportunities throughout the appraisal process;

- implementation of an appeals procedure;

- frequent and close collaboration with external review bodies, such as the NCCs, TACs and the Royal Colleges.

NICE's engagement with a broad representation of stakeholders, from multiple sectors and disciplines, introduces a variety of perspectives into the appraisal and decision-making process. This is particularly helpful when reaching consensus on conflicting evidence or recommendations that require knowledge of both scientific literature and the realities of clinical practice. Moreover, given the paucity of scientific evidence about patient treatment preferences and viewpoints on issues such as equity and fairness in health care, it is important to elicit such perspectives from a variety of stakeholders. At implementation, a high level of stakeholder involvement increases public and professional ownership in the guidance, thereby enhancing the likelihood that it will guide effective decision-making and clinical practice.

The methods that NICE employs or promulgates have both advantages and drawbacks. In general, methods are transparent and standardized across appraisals. The transparency of the nomination and decision-making process for topic selection has improved recently, but NICE has focused mainly on new technologies, rather than those in practice. Consequently, it is likely that a number of cost-ineffective therapies are employed currently within the NHS. STAs raise further questions about topic prioritization as the criteria for their selection are not always clear.

NICE commonly assesses technologies (primarily drugs) in the same class. While this can produce greater efficiency and comparability across similar products, often it is associated with problems resulting from a lack of head-to-head studies and pressurizes manufacturers to demonstrate additional benefits in order to justify a premium price (Drummond, 2006). The latter is also true of STAs as these place more emphasis on analyses submitted by the manufacturer and less on external review. However, unlike assessments across product class, STAs are usually most appropriate in situations where there are a limited number of comparators.

Within the appraisal process, the NICE approach has the potential drawback of unnecessary duplication of effort. Manufacturers and the academic (TAR) group often work in apparent isolation so difficulties may ensue if conflicts surrounding the available evidence are resolved late in the appraisal process. Moreover, the time frame between the announcement of a topic and the commencement of the review process (typically, several months) may render it difficult for stakeholders to assemble appropriate evidence. Key questions within the assessment may not be made clear until the project scope is finalized. Furthermore, a lengthy preliminary process may impose time pressures on the relevant groups and stakeholders towards the end of the appraisal process. The time frame permits new information to be incorporated towards the end of the process without necessarily allowing time for review and critical appraisal. It is important that NICE balances transparency and collective participation with efficiency.

Gafni and Birch (2004) question NICE's methods for considering resource allocation. In particular, issues of efficient and equitable resource use cannot be addressed, because the costs and health benefits of a technology are reviewed without examining the associated opportunity costs. Failure to consider such costs (and where to disinvest) within the assessment process (and subsequent decisions) may lead to increases in NHS expenditure without evidence of health gain; greater inequalities in access to services; and problems for the sustainability of public funding for new technologies. As NICE does not consider affordability when making judgments about CE (i.e. an intervention that the NHS cannot afford may be deemed cost-effective by NICE), government mechanisms should be put in place to respond to such circumstances. That said, the DH recognizes that NICE has a key role in advising on areas of disinvestment or obsolete technologies, and is exploring means of identifying topics for such evaluations.

NICE has served as a model for methodological development and spurred growth in new assessment approaches (e.g. probabilistic models). This is aided by steady funding for training fellowships (e.g. via NHS R&D) and the recruitment of skilled health economic personnel.

Implementation can either hinder or facilitate the effective use of NICE's recommendations. There does not appear to be stringent implementation of guidance, but there is some evidence of influence, such as the mandated three-month requirement. However, a significant hurdle to effective implementation is securing the funding to offer recommended technologies and interventions within a resource-constrained environment. In addition, restrictions in use frequently pose challenge to implementation, as certain patient populations or indications may have limited access to a technology.

A recent study found mixed implementation of NICE guidance, by technology and location (Sheldon et al., 2004). For example, the use of orlistats and taxanes grew rapidly following publication of guidance, although compliance among Trusts appeared to be inconsistent across a range of guidelines. Compliance is likely to depend upon the Trusts preparedness (through established structures and processes) to manage implementation of NICE guidance. Sheldon et al. (2004) suggest that implementation is likely to improve if the guidance is clear and based on an understanding of clinical practice and/or the policy process; and well-supported in terms of funding and professional involvement. Moreover, the credibility of NICE guidance is dependent on the transparency of the relevant committee's decision-making process. It is crucial that such decisions are consistent across the broad range of appraisals undertaken on health technologies and interventions, and that the views of consultees are taken sufficiently into account. The application of a coherent and explicit approach is necessary for NICE to achieve the central objectives of the NHS.

Table A6.2. *Overview of HTA governance, processes and role in decision-making in the United Kingdom*

United Kingdom	
HTA governance & organization	
Institutions/committees	NICE, NHS Centre for Reviews and Dissemination, NCCHTA.
	Other entities involved in HTA: academia, the DH, UK Cochrane Centre, UK National Screening Committee and the corporate sector.
Entities responsible for reviewing HTA evidence for priority-setting and decision-making	DH.
	NICE: Advisory Committee/Programme Development Group (public health); Appraisal Committee (health technology); Advisory Committee (interventions); and Guideline Development Group (clinical guidelines).
HTA agenda-setting body(s)	Primarily DH in collaboration with NICE.
Areas for HTA	Medicines, medical devices, diagnostic techniques, surgical procedures and health prevention/promotion activities.

(cont.)

Table A6.2. *(cont.)*

Reimbursement requirements and limitations	Not relevant.
Stakeholder involvement	Broad participation from a variety of stakeholders – health professionals, patient groups, general public, manufacturers, professional associations, methodological experts, etc.
International collaboration	EuroScan, HTAi, HEN, EUnetHTA, INAHTA and G-I-N.

HTA topic selection & analytical design

Governance of topic selection	NICE topic selection consideration panels, Minister of Health, DH.
Criteria for topic selection	• burden of disease (population affected, morbidity, mortality);
	• resource impact (cost impact on NHS or public sector);
	• clinical and policy importance (whether topic is within a government priority area);
	• presence of inappropriate variation(s) in practice;
	• potential factors affecting the timeliness of the guidance to be produced (degree of urgency, relevancy of guideline at expected date of delivery);
	• likelihood of guidance having an impact on public health and quality of life, reduction in health inequalities, or the delivery of quality programmes or interventions.
	• Also, appropriateness and NICE's ability to commence development of a guideline.

Criteria for assessment	Strength of the available evidence (nature, quality and degree of uncertainty), importance of outcomes, health impact, CE, inequalities, feasibility of implementation, impact on the NHS, acceptability, broad clinical and government policy priorities, health need.
Criteria outlined or publicly-available	Yes.
Analysis perspective	For reference cases: NHS and PSS (personal social services). In non-reference cases: societal, not including productivity costs.
Duration required to conduct assessments	Interventional guidance: ~46 weeks.
	Technology appraisals: ~51 weeks (MTAs); ~32 weeks (STAs).
	Clinical guidelines: ~72 weeks.
	Short clinical guidelines: ~40 weeks.

Evidence requirements & assessment methods[67]

Documents required from manufacturer	Complete list of all studies concerning the technology under review; executive summary of not more than 5 pages; main submission of not more than 50 pages, which should include:
	(1) aims of treatment and current approved indications
	(2) assessment of clinical effectiveness
	(3) assessment of CE
	(4) assessment of resource impact on the NHS, uptake/treatment rates, population health gain, resource implications and financial costs
	(5) data appendix
	(6) electronic copy of any model used in the CE analysis, if applicable.

(cont.)

---

67. Section applies primarily to NICE.

Table A6.2. *(cont.)*

Systematic literature review and synthesis	Health effects should be identified and quantified, and all data sources described clearly. Synthesis of outcome data through meta-analysis is appropriate, provided there are sufficient relevant and valid data using comparable outcome measures.
Unpublished data/ grey literature	Not routine.
Preferred clinical study type/ evidence	Prefer prospective RCTs with a naturalistic design. Effectiveness is preferred over efficacy, especially long-term effectiveness.
Type of economic assessment preferred or required	CE or cost-utility analysis. Health effects should be expressed in terms of QALYs. Cost-benefit analysis may be used in specific situations. In addition, cost-consequence approach may be adopted to take account of the complex and multidimensional character of public health interventions and programmes. Issues such as equity and distribution can also inform the analysis.
Availability of guidelines outlining methodological requirements	Published by NICE.
Choice of comparator	Current best alternative care or alternative therapies routinely used in the NHS.
Specification of outcome variable	Mortality, morbidity, quality of life, willingness to pay (in some situations).
Sub-group analyses	Yes, especially high-risk patients.
Costs included in analysis	Direct costs, but those that refer to the NHS and PSS. May also add travel and other public-sector costs, but typically does not include productivity costs.

Incremental analyses required	Yes.
Time horizon	Period over which main differences between technologies and their likely health effects and use of health-care resources are expected to be experienced.
Equity issues	An additional QALY has the same weight regardless of the other characteristics of the individual receiving the health benefit.
Discounting	Base case: 3.5% (health effects and costs); sensitivity analysis: varies between 0%-6% (health effects and costs). For manufacturer submissions: base case: 6% (costs), 1.5% (benefits); sensitivity analysis: 6% (costs), varies between 0%-6% (health effects).
Modelling	Modelling is typically required. May be decision-analytical model using aggregated data or statistical model using patient-level data.
Sensitivity analyses	Probabilistic sensitivity analysis. All data sources must be justified and point estimates, ranges and distribution of values identified to test best- and worst-case scenarios.
CE or willingness-to-pay threshold	No fixed threshold, but evidence suggests that NICE employs a range of £20 000/QALY to £40 000/QALY. NICE primarily bases decisions on incremental CE ratios below £20 000/QALY. NICE may accept higher thresholds, but additional justification is required (e.g. innovative nature of technology, equity, public health necessity).
Missing or incomplete data	Not available.
Support for methodological development	Yes.

(cont.)

Table A6.2. *(cont.)*

HTA dissemination & implementation

Channels for HTA results dissemination	NICE web site, publications, international HTA organizations, media, dissemination/ implementation tools provided to stakeholders (via NICE web site).
Use of HTA results	To develop standards; guide patient-care decisions; inform strategies to meet government indicators and targets; support decision-making on NHS funding and resource allocation; guide education and training of health professionals.
Evidence considered in decision-making	See HTA topic selection and analytical design section.
Any reported obstacles to effective implementation	Insufficient funding, lack of support from health professionals; inadequate structure to support implementation amongst the Trusts; duplication of effort during appraisal process, timelines, etc.
Formal processes to measure impact	Yes.
Processes for re-evaluation or appeals	Re-evaluation every 4 years (NICE technology appraisals); 4-6 years (NICE clinical guidelines); 3 years (NICE public health guidance); 1-5 years (STAs). NICE incorporates a formal appeals process.
Accountability for stakeholder input	Several opportunities for stakeholder submission of evidence, review and comment.
Transparent/public decision-making process	Information on most appraisal and decision-making processes is publicly available via the NICE web site.

Sources: Zentner et al., 2005; OECD, 2003; NICE, 2006 (a-e); NICE, 2004 (a-g).

REFERENCES

AdvaMed. *Technology assessment by public and private payers*. Washington D.C. Advanced Medical Technology Association, 2000.

Anell A. Priority setting for pharmaceuticals. *European Journal of Health Economics*, 2004, 5: 28-35.

Anell A, Persson U. Reimbursement and clinical guidance for pharmaceuticals in Sweden. *European Journal of Health Economics*, 2005, 14(S1): S237-254.

Anell A, Svarvar P. Pharmacoeconomics and clinical practice guidelines: A survey of attitudes in Swedish formulary committees. *Pharmacoeconomics*, 2000, 17(2):175-85.

Asch SM, Sloss EM, Hogan C, Brook RH, Kravitz RL. Measuring underuse and necessary care among elderly Medicare beneficiaries using inpatient and outpatient claims. *JAMA*. 2000, 284:2325-33.

Banta D. The development of health technology assessment. *Health Policy*, 2003, 63:121-132.

Banta D, Oortwijn W. Health technology assessment and health care in the European Union. *International Journal of Technology Assessment in Health Care*, 2000, 16(2):626-635.

Barbieri M et al. Variability in cost-effectiveness estimates for pharmaceuticals in western Europe: lessons for inferring generalizability. *Value in Health*, 2005, 8(1):10-23.

Battista R, Hodge MJ. The evolving paradigm of health technology assessment: reflections for the Millennium. *Journal of the Canadian Medical Association*, 1999, 160(10):1464-1467.

Bell CM et al. Bias in published cost-effectiveness studies: a systematic review. *BMJ*, 2006, 332:699-703.

Bellanger M, Cherilova V, Paris V. The health benefit basket in France. *European Journal of Health Economics,* 2005, 6(Suppl.1):24-29.

Berg M, van der Grinten T, Klazinga N. Technology assessment, priority setting and appropriate care in Dutch health care. *International Journal of Health Technology Assessment*, 2004, 20(1):35-43.

Bos M. Health technology assessment in the Netherlands. *International Journal of Health Technology Assessment*, 2000, 16(2):485-519.

Boulenger S et al. Can economic evaluations be made more transferable? *European Journal of Health Economics*, 2005, 6:334-346.

Brownman GP. Development and aftercare of clinical guidelines: the balance between rigor and pragmatism. *JAMA*, 2001, 286:1509-1511.

Busse R, Riesberg A. *Health care systems in transition: Germany*. Copenhagen, WHO Regional Office for Europe on behalf of the European Observatory on Health Systems and Policies, 2004.

Busse R et al. Best practice in undertaking and reporting health technology assessments. *International Journal of Health Technology Assessment*, 2002, 18:361-422.

Busse R et al. *Determining the "health benefit basket" of the statutory health insurance scheme in Germany*. European Journal of Health Economics, 2005, 6(Suppl 1):30-36.

Cairns J. Providing guidance to the NHS: the Scottish Medicines Consortium and the National Institute for Clinical Excellence compared. *Health Policy*, 2006, 76(2):134-143.

Carlsson P. Health technology assessment and priority setting for health policy in Sweden. *International Journal of Health Technology Assessment*, 2004, 20(1):44-54.

Carlsson P, Hultin H, Tornwall J. The early experiences of a national system for the identification and assessment of emerging health care technologies in Sweden. *International Journal of Health Technology Assessment*, 1998, 14(4):687-694.

Carlsson P, Jorgensen T. Scanning the horizon for emerging health technologies: conclusions from a European workshop. *International Journal of Technology Assessment in Health Care*, 1998, 14(4):695-704.

Carlsson P et al. Health technology assessment in Sweden. *International Journal of Health Technology Assessment*, 2000, 16:560-575.

Cookson R, Maynard A. Health technology assessment in Europe. Improving clarity and performance. *International Journal of Health Technology Assessment*, 2000, 16(2):639-650.

Coulter A. Perspectives on health technology assessment: response from the patient's perspective. *International Journal of Health Technology Assessment*, 2004, 20(1):92-96.

Council for Public Health and Health Care. *Sensible and sustainable care.* Recommendations by the Council for Public Health and Health Care to the Minister of Health, Welfare and Sport, 2006 (http://www.rvz.net/data/download/Advies–DenZ–samenvatting–engels.doc).

Culyer AJ. NICE´s use of cost effectiveness as an exemplar of a deliberative process. *Health Economics, Policy and Law*, 2006, 1:299-318.

Cutler D, McClellan M. Is technological change in medicine worth it? *Health Affairs*, 2001, 20: 11-29.

den Exter A et al. *Health care systems in transition: Netherlands.* Copenhagen, WHO Regional Office for Europe on behalf of the European Observatory on Health Systems and Policies, 2004.

Department of Health. *The new NHS: modern, dependable.* London, HMSO, 1997.

Department of Health. *The NHS plan: a plan for investment, a plan for reform.* London, The Stationery Office Limited, 2000.

Devlin N, Parkin D. Does NICE have a cost-effectiveness threshold and what other factors influence its decisions? A binary choice analysis. *Health Economics*, 2004, 13:437-452.

Deyo RA. Cascade effects of medical technology. *Annual Review Public Health*. 2002, 23:23-44.

Douw K, Vondeling H, Eskildensen D, Simpson S. Use of the Internet in scanning the horizon for new and emerging health technologies: a survey of agencies involved in horizon scanning. *Journal of Medical Internet Research*, 2003; 5(1):e6.

Douw K, Vonderling H. Selection of new health technologies for assessment aimed at horizon scanning systems. *International Journal of Health Technology Assessment*, 2006, 22(2):177-183.

Draborg E, Andersen CK. What influences the choice of assessment methods in health technology assessments? Statistical analysis of international health technology assessments from 1989 to 2002. *International Journal of Health Technology Assessment*, 2005, 22:19-25.

Draborg E, Andersen CK. Recommendations in health technology assessments worldwide. *International Journal of Health Technology Assessment*, 2006, 22(2):155-160.

Draborg E et al. International comparisons of the definition and the practical application of health technology assessment. *International Journal of Health Technology Assessment*, 2005, 21:89-95.

Drummond M. The use of economic evidence by healthcare decision makers. *European Journal of Health Economics*, 2001, 2:2-3.

Drummond M. Making economic evaluations more accessible to health care decision-makers. *European Journal of Health Economics* 2003;4: 246-247.

Drummond M. *Health technology assessment. Has the UK got it right?*, London School of Economics, 2006 (Merck Trust Lecture 2005/2006).

Drummond M, Weatherly H. Implementing the findings of health technology assessments: if the CAT got out of the bag, can the TAIL wag the dog? *International Journal of Technology Assessment in Health Care*, 2000, 16(1):1-12.

Eisenberg JM. Ten lessons for evidence-based technology assessment. *JAMA*, 1999, 17:1865-1869.

Eisenberg JM, Zarin D. Health technology assessment in the United States: past, present, and future. *International Journal of Health Technology Assessment in Health Care*, 2002, 18:192-198.

Eskola J et al. *The future of FinOHTA: an external review.* Helsinki, FinOHTA, 2004 (Report 23).

European Collaboration for Health Technology Assessment Project. Working Group 6 Report. *International Journal of Health Technology Assessment in Health Care*, 2002, 18 (2):447-455.

European Commission. *Inventory of Community and Member States' incentive measures to aid the research, marketing, development and availability of orphan medicinal products,* 2006 (http://ec.europa.eu/enterprise/pharmaceuticals/ orphanmp/doc/inventory–2006–08.pdf).

FinOHTA (2006a). [web site]. Helsinki, FinOHTA (www.finohta.stakes.fi).

FinOHTA (2006b). *Impakti.* Vol.2. Helsinki, FinOHTA, 2006.

Fleurette F, Banta D. Health technology assessment in France. *International Journal of Health Technology Assessment in Health Care*, 2000, 16: 400-411.

Gafni A, Birch ST. The NICE reference case requirement: more pain for what, if any, gain? *PharmacoEconomics*, 2004, 22(4):271-273.

Garber AM. Advances in cost-effectiveness analysis of health interventions. In: Culyer AJ and Newhouse JP, eds *Handbook of health economics*, Vol. 1. Amsterdam North-Holland, 2000: 181-221.

Garcia-Altes A, Ondategui-Parra S, Neumann P. Cross-national comparison of technology assessment processes. *International Journal of Health Technology Assessment in Health Care*, 2004, 20(3):300-310.

Gibis B, Koch-Wulkan PW, Bultman J. Shifting criteria for benefit decisions in social health insurance systems. In: Saltman RB, Busse R, Figueras J, eds. *Social health insurance systems in western Europe.* Copenhagen, WHO Regional Office for Europe on behalf of the European Observatory on Health Systems and Policies, 2004.

Glenngard AH, Hjalte, F, Svensson, M, Anell, A, and Bankauskaite V. *Health care systems in transition: Sweden.* Copenhagen, WHO Regional Office for Europe on behalf of the European Observatory on Health Systems and Policies, 2005.

Goddard M et al. Priority-setting in health – a political economy perspective. *Health Economics, Policy, and Law*, 2006, 1:79-90.

Goodman CS. Healthcare technology assessment: methods, framework, and role in policy making. *American Journal of Managed Care*, 1998, 4:SP200-214.

Greenberg D, Winkelmayer WC, Neumann PJ. Prevailing judgments about society's willingness to pay for QALY or life-year gained. *International Journal of Public Health*, 2005, 2(Suppl.1):301.

Grol R, Grimshaw J. Evidence-based implementation of evidence-based medicine. *Joint Commission Journal on Quality Improvement*, 1999, 25:503-513.

Hagenfeldt K et al. Systems for routine information sharing in HTA: working group 2 report. *International Journal of Technology Assessment in Health Care*, 2002, 18:273-320.

Hailey D, Cowley DE, Dankiw W. The impact of health technology assessment. *Community Health Studies*, 1990, 14(3):223-234.

Hailey D et al. The use and impact of rapid health technology assessments. *International Journal of Technology Assessment in Health Care*, 2000, 16(2):651-656.

Health Council of the Netherlands. *From implementation to learning: the importance of a two-way dialogue between practice and science in health care.* The Hague, Health Council of the Netherlands, 2000.

Health Council of the Netherlands: work programme 2006. The Hague, Health Council of the Netherlands, 2005 (Publication no. A05/05E, RGO publication no. 50E).

Health Council of the Netherlands. *Network.* The Hague, Health Council of the Netherlands, 2006, Vol 21:No. 2.

Henshall C et al. Priority-setting for health technology assessment. Theoretical considerations and practical approaches. Priority-setting subgroup of the EUR-ASSESS Project. *International Journal of Technology Assessment in Health Care*, 1997, 13:144-185.

Henshall C et al. Health technology assessment in policy and practice. Working group 6 report. *International Journal of Health Technology Assessment*, 2002, 18(2):447-455.

Hjelmgren J, Berggren F, Andersson F. Health economic guidelines – similarities, differences, and some implications. *Value Health*, 2001, 4(3):225-250.

Hutton J et al. Framework for describing and classifying decision-making systems using technology assessment to determine the reimbursement of health technologies (fourth hurdle systems). *International Journal of Technology Assessment in Health Care*, 2006, 21(1):10-18.

ISPOR. *Country-specific pharmacoeconomic guidelines.* Lawrenceville, NJ, USA, International Society for Pharmacoeconomics and Outcomes Research 1999 (available at: http://www.ispor.org/PEguidelines/COUNTRYSPECIFIC.asp, accessed 1 October 2007).

Jacob R, McGregor M. Assessing the impact of health technology assessment. *International Journal of Technology Assessment in Health Care*, 1997, 13(1): 68-80.

Jarvelin J. *Health care systems in transition: Finland.* Copenhagen, WHO Regional Office for Europe on behalf of the European Observatory on Health Systems and Policies, 2002.

Jonsson E. Development of health technology assessment in Europe. *International Journal of Technology Assessment in Health Care*, 2002, 18: 171–183.

Jonsson E, Banta HD. Management of health technologies: an international view. *BMJ*, 1999, 319:1293.

Lauslahti K et al. Health technology assessment in Finland. *International Journal of Technology Assessment in Health Care*, 2000, 16:382-399.

Mason A, Smith P. *Health basket project benefit report: England.* Brussels, European Health Management Association, 2005.

Maynard A, McDaid D. ASTEC: the implications for policy makers. In: Cookson R et al., eds. *Analysis of the scientific and technical evaluation of health-care interventions in the European Union. Report to the European Commission, 2000.* London, LSE Health and Social Care, 2000 (www.lse.ac.uk/Depts/lsehsc/astec–report.htm, accessed 1 October 2007).

Maynard A, McDaid D. Evaluating health interventions. Exploiting the potential. *Health Policy*, 2003, 63:215-226.

McEwan A. Does health technology assessment put patient care at risk? *Journal of Nuclear Medicine*, 2005, 46(12):1939.

McGregor M, Brophy JM. End-user involvement in health technology assessment (HTA) development: a way to increase impact. *International Journal of Health Technology Assessment*, 2005, 21:263-267.

McNeil BJ. Hidden barriers to improvement in the quality of care. *New England Journal of Medicine*, 2001; 345: 1612-20.

Michaels J. Improving NICE's social value judgements. *BMJ*, 2006, 332:48-50.

National Institute for Clinical Excellence. *Guide to the technology appraisal process.* London, NICE, 2004a.

National Institute for Clinical Excellence. *About the citizens council.* London, NICE, 2004b (http://www.nice.org.uk/page.aspx?o=113692, accessed 1 October 2007).

National Institute for Clinical Excellence. *Guide to the methods of technology appraisal.* London, NICE, 2004c.

National Institute for Clinical Excellence. *Contributing to a technology appraisal: a guide for manufacturers and sponsors.* London, NICE, 2004d.

National Institute for Clinical Excellence. *Contributing to a technology appraisal: a guide for patient/carer groups.* London, NICE, 2004e.

National Institute for Clinical Excellence. *Appraisal process: guidance for appellants.* London, NICE, 2004f.

National Institute for Clinical Excellence. *The interventional procedures programme.* London, NICE, 2004g.

National Institute for Clinical Excellence. *Methods for the development of NICE public health guidance.* London, NICE, 2006a.

National Institute for Clinical Excellence. *Department of Health selection criteria.* London, NICE, 2006b (http://www.nice.org.uk/364841, accessed 1 October 2007).

National Institute for Clinical Excellence. *Guide to the single technology (STA) process.* London, NICE, 2006c.

National Institute for Clinical Excellence. *The guidelines manual.* London, NICE, 2006d.

National Institute for Clinical Excellence. *The guideline development process: an overview for stakeholders, the public and the NHS (2nd edition).* London, NICE, 2006e.

National Institute for Clinical Excellence. *Putting NICE guidance into practice.* London, NICE, 2006f.

NCCHTA. About the HTA programme. London, Department of Health, 2006 (http://www.hta.nhsweb.nhs.uk/about/index.shtml., accessed 1 October 2007).

Neumann J. *Using cost-effectiveness analysis to improve heath care: opportunities and barriers.* New York, Oxford University Press, 2004.

Neumann J et al. Growth and quality of the cost-utility literature, 1976-2001. *Value Health*, 2005, 8:3-9.

Newdick C. Evaluating new health technology in the English national health service. In: Jost TS, ed. *Health care coverage: an international comparative study.* Maidenhead, Berkshire, Open University Press, 2005.

Newhouse JP. Medical care costs: how much welfare loss? *Journal of Economic Perspectives*, 1992, 6:3-21.

Oliver A, Mossialos E, Robinson R. Health technology assessment and its influence on health-care priority setting. *International Journal of Health Technology Assessment*, 2004, 20(1):1-10.

Oortwijn WJ et al. Identification and priority-setting for health technology assessment in the Netherlands: actors and activities. *Health Policy*, 1999, 47:241-253.

Oortwijn WJ et al. Priority setting for health technology assessment in the Netherlands: principles and practice. *Health Policy*, 2002, 62(3):227-242.

Organisation for Economic Co-operation and Development. *OECD heath data: a comparative analysis of 30 OECD countries.* Paris, OECD, 2002.

Organisation for Economic Co-operation and Development. *Survey of pharmacoeconomic assessment in eleven countries.* Paris, OECD, 2003 (OECD Working Papers No. 4).

Organisation for Economic Co-operation and Development. *Health technologies and decision-making.* Paris, OECD, 2005.

Orvain J, Xerri B, Matillon Y. Overview of health technology assessment in France. *International Journal of Health Technology Assessment*, 2003, 20(1): 25-34.

Paolucci F, Scout F, van de Ven W. *Economic rationales for the design of health care financing schemes.* Oslo, Health Organization Research Norway (HORN), 2006 (Working paper 2006:3).

Perleth M, Busse R. Health technology assessment in Germany. *International Journal of Health Technology Assessment*, 2000, 16:412-428.

Perry S, Tharner M. Medical innovation and the critical role of health technology assessment. *JAMA*, 1999, 282:1869-1872.

Pharmaceutical Benefits Board. *Act (2002:160) on Pharmaceutical Benefits, etc.* Solna, Pharmaceutical Benefits Board (http://www.lfn.se/upload/English/ENG_Act_2002-160.pdf).

Pharma Industry Finland. *Situation report.* Helsinki, PIF newsletter, 2: May 2004.

Rasanen P et al. Use of quality-adjusted life years for the estimation of effectiveness in health care: a systematic literature review. *International Journal of Health Technology Assessment*, 2006, 20:67-70.

Rawlins MD, Culyer AJ. National Institute for Clinical Excellence and its value judgments. *BMJ*, 2004, 329:224-227.

Rotstein D, Laupacis A. Differences between systematic reviews and health technology assessments: a trade-off between the ideals of scientific rigor and the realities of policy making. *International Journal of Health Technology Assessment*, 2004, 20:177-183.

Rutten F. Health technology assessment and policy from the economic perspective. *International Journal of Health Technology Assessment*, 2004, 22(2):235-241.

Rutten F, Brouwer W, Niessen L. Practice guidelines based on clinical and economic evidence. *European Journal of Health Economics*, 2005, 6:91-93.

Sandier S, Paris V, Polton D. *Health systems in transition: France.* In: Thompson S, Mossialos E, eds. Copenhagen, WHO Regional Office for Europe on behalf of the European Observatory on Health Systems and Policies, 2004.

Sassi F. Setting priorities for the evaluation of health interventions: when theory does not meet practice. *Health Policy*, 2003, 63:141-154.

SBU, 2006. Stockholm, Swedish Council on Technology Assessment in Health Care (http://www.sbu.se/www/index.asp).

Schwappach DL. Resource allocation, social values, and the QALY: a review of the debate and empirical evidence. *Health Expect*ations, 2002, 5(3):210-222.

Schreyogg J et al. Defining the "health benefit basket" in nine European countries. *European Journal of Health Economics*, 2005, Suppl 1(6):2-10.

Sheingold SH. Technology assessment, coverage decisions, and conflict: the role of guidelines. *American Journal of Managed Care*, 2005, 4:SP117-25.

Sheldon TA et al. What's the evidence that NICE guidance has been implemented? Results from a national evaluation using time series analysis, audit of patients' notes, and interviews. *BMJ*, 2004, 329:999 (doi:10.1136/BMJ.329.7473.999).

Stevens A, Milne R. Health technology assessment in England and Wales. *International Journal of Health Technology Assessment*, 2004, 20(1):11-24.

Stolk EA, Poley MJ. Criteria for determining a basic health services package: recent development in the Netherlands. *European Journal of Health Economics*, 2005, 50:2-7.

Stolk EA, Rutten F. *The health basket in the Netherlands.* Rotterdam, Institute for Medical Technology Assessment, 2005 (Report no. 05.75).

Swedish Council on Technology Assessment in Health Care (2007) [web site]. Stockholm (http://www.sbu.se/en/).

Taylor R. Pharmaceutical regulation: the early experiences of the NHS National Institute for Clinical Excellence (NICE) appraisal process – where are we heading? *Value Health*, 2001, 4:8-11.

Taylor R et al. Inclusion of cost-effectiveness in licensing requirements for new drugs: a fourth hurdle. *BMJ*, 2004, 329:972-975.

Towse A. The efficient use of pharmaceuticals: does Europe have any lessons for a Medicare drug benefit? *Health Affairs*, 2003, 22(3):42-45.

United Kingdom House of Commons (2007). Written answers. London, Hansard (http://www.publications.parliament.uk/pa/cm200607/cmhansrd/cm070723/text/70723w0046.htm).

United Kingdom National Health Service (2003). R&D Health Technology Assessment Programme, 2003 (http://www.hta.nhsweb.nhs.uk/about/index.shtml).

Van Oostenbruggen MF et al. Penny and pound wise. Pharmacoeconomics from a governmental perspective. *Pharmacoeconomics*, 2005, 23:219–226.

Velasco Garrido, M, Busse, R. *Health Technology Assessment—An Introduction on Objectives, Role of Evidence, and Structure in Europe.* Policy Brief. Brussels, European Observatory on Health Systems and Policies, 2005.

Williams AH, Crookson RA. Equity-efficiency trade-offs in health technology assessment. *International Journal of Health Technology Assessment*, 2006, 22(1):1-9.

Woolf S, Henshall C. Health technology assessment in the United Kingdom. *International Journal of Health Technology Assessment*, 2000, 16:591-625.

Zentner A, Valasco-Garrido M, Busse R. Methods for the comparative evaluation of pharmaceuticals. *GMS Health Technology Assessment*, 2005, 1:Doc09.